The Anti -
Inflammatory Diet
for Beginners

A Super-Easy Guide with 100+ Wholesome Recipes with

Natural Ingredients and Special Diet Options.

Includes an efficient 4-Week Meal Plan

By

SOPHIA WELLS

SCROLL TO THE END AND SCAN THE QR CODES TO PRINT: The Quick Reference Guides & The Grocery List

Nourish and Heal your body with the transformative **power of food!**

This cookbook is much more than just a collection of recipes. It's a complete guide to embracing self-care at 365 degrees. Inside you'll find over 100 nutritious and natural recipes designed to support your journey to optimal health.

These recipes will empower you to take control of your health, enjoy delicious, nutritious meals, and cultivate a deeper sense of well-being. A 4 week meal plan will help you to feel more confident.

Embark on this journey to a healthier, happier you and let every meal nourish and heal your body and soul.

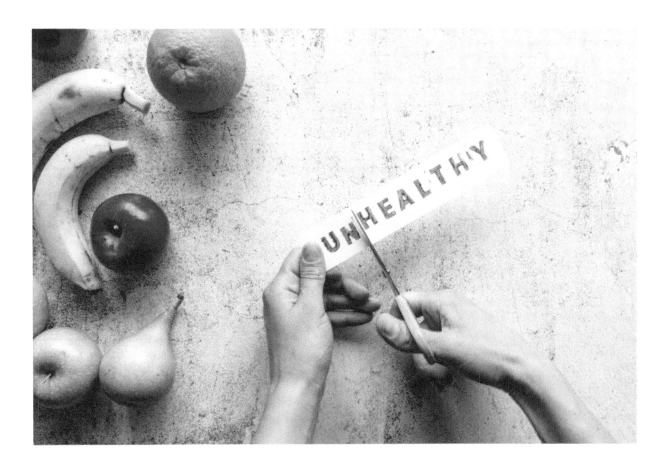

TABLE OF CONTENTS

INTRODUCTION

Dear Reader,

Welcome to "The Anti-Inflammatory Diet": A must-have treasure trove of delicious health and self-care recipes

I am Sophia Wells, a dietitian, nutritionist, and chef, and I am excited to share with you this journey into natural health and wellness.

I have always believed in the power of food as a natural medicine. My clients have experienced remarkable improvements in their health, from increased energy levels to improved overall well-being.

Inspired by these positive changes, I felt compelled to create this cookbook to share with you a natural and healthy way to nourish our bodies and our well-being.

This book is more than a collection of recipes-it is a guide to a holistic lifestyle that promotes health and vitality.

What You Will Discover

1. **Wholesome Recipes:** A diverse selection of recipes that prioritize natural ingredients and avoid artificial additives. These recipes are crafted to be both delicious and nutritious, helping you to enjoy the process of eating healthy.

2. **Natural Remedies:** Insights into the medicinal properties of various ingredients, showing you how food can be used as medicine. Learn about natural remedies for common ailments and how to incorporate them into your diet.

3. **Mindful Eating:** Tips on how to practice mindful eating, encouraging you to savor your food and listen to your body's needs. Mindful eating is a key component of self-care and overall wellness.

4. **Self-Care Practices:** Beyond recipes, this cookbook includes self-care routines and practices that complement a healthy diet. Discover ways to integrate self-care into your daily life, enhancing both your physical and mental well-being.

Embarking on a journey to natural health is a commitment to nurturing your body and mind. This cookbook is here to support you every step of the way, offering practical advice and inspiring you to embrace a lifestyle that promotes vitality and longevity.

PRINCIPLES OF A HEALTHY AND ANTI-INFLAMMATORY DIET

The body possesses an innate ability to heal itself when provided with the right conditions.

- **The Body's Innate Healing Ability:** The human body is designed to heal itself. By giving the correct foods to our bodies, we create an optimal internal environment to facilitate this natural process.

- **Holistic Approach**: It is essential to address the root causes of health problems, rather than just treating the symptoms. This holistic perspective considers physical, emotional and environmental factors.

- **Supportive Environment**: Factors such as proper nutrition, adequate hydration, regular exercise, and mental well-being are crucial for maintaining a body that can heal and sustain itself.

- **Importance of Diet in Health:** What we eat directly affects our overall well-being and our ability to heal.

- **Whole Foods**: "The Anti-Inflammatory Diet" promotes a diet rich in whole foods, including fresh fruits, vegetables, whole grains, nuts and seeds. These foods provide essential nutrients that support bodily functions and promote healing

- **Natural Ingredients**: Avoiding processed foods and artificial additives is a fundamental principle. Natural, unprocessed foods are better recognized and utilized by the body, resulting in better health outcomes.

- **Balanced Nutrition**: Ensuring a balance of macronutrients-carbohydrates, proteins and fats-is critical. This book emphasizes the importance of consuming these nutrients in their healthiest forms, such as complex carbohydrates, lean proteins and healthy fats.

- **Hydration and Detoxification:** Proper hydration and detoxification are other critical and substantial aspects. This diet highlights the importance of water and natural detoxification methods to maintain the health of the body. Drinking adequate amounts of clean, filtered water is essential. Staying hydrated helps eliminate toxins, supports metabolic processes, and maintains cell health.

- **Detoxification**: Natural detox methods, including consuming detoxifying foods (like leafy greens and certain fruits) and practices (like intermittent fasting), are recommended to cleanse the body of harmful substances.

- **Plant-Based Nutrition:** While not strictly advocating vegetarianism or veganism, this diet is predominantly plant-based. Plant-based foods are rich in nutrients and promote optimal health.

- **Vegetables and Fruits**: A diverse intake of fruits and vegetables provides a wide range of vitamins, minerals and antioxidants. It is recommended to consume these foods in abundance to support immune function and overall health.

- **Legumes and Nuts**: They are important sources of protein, fiber and healthy fats. It is essential to incorporate a variety of legumes and nuts into the diet to meet nutritional needs.

- **Mindful Eating Practices**
  It is also important how you eat, not just what you eat. Mindful eating practices can improve digestion and overall meal satisfaction.

1. **Eating Slowly**: Taking time to eat and chew food properly aids digestion and allows the body to better absorb nutrients.

2. **Listening to the Body**: pay attention to hunger and fullness cues, which can prevent overeating and promote a healthy relationship with food.

3. **Regular Meal Times**: Maintaining regular meal times helps regulate metabolism and ensures consistent energy levels throughout the day.

4. **Avoiding Harmful Substances** that can be detrimental to health, including processed sugars, artificial sweeteners, trans fats, and excessive caffeine and alcohol. Processed Foods: These often contain additives and preservatives that can disrupt bodily functions and lead to health issues.

It is recommended to use natural sweeteners such as honey or stevia in moderation and to choose healthy fats from sources such as avocados and nuts.

Importance of diet in achieving and maintaining optimal health

A well-balanced, nutrient-dense diet provides the foundation for achieving and maintaining optimal health.

A nutritious diet is fundamental to health, providing essential macronutrients and micronutrients that support the body's functions.

1. **Macronutrients**:

   o **Carbohydrates**: Complex carbohydrates, found in whole grains, vegetables, and legumes, provide sustained energy and are crucial for digestive health due to their fiber content.

   o **Proteins**: Essential for building and repairing tissues, proteins also play a key role in immune function and the production of enzymes and hormones. Sources such as beans, lentils, nuts, seeds, and lean meats are particularly beneficial.

   o **Fats**: Healthy fats, including those from avocados, nuts, seeds, and olive oil, are vital for brain health, hormone production, and maintaining cellular integrity.

2. **Micronutrients**:

   • **Vitamins and Minerals**: These are required in smaller amounts but are critical for disease prevention and overall health. For example, vitamin C is essential for immune function, while calcium and vitamin D are crucial for bone health.

Diet and Disease Prevention

A nutrient-rich diet is instrumental in preventing chronic diseases.

• **Heart Disease**: Diets high in fruits, vegetables, whole grains, and lean proteins help lower cholesterol levels, reduce blood pressure, and improve heart health. The antioxidants and fiber in these foods play a significant role in preventing cardiovascular disease.
• **Diabetes**: A balanced diet that includes whole grains, fiber, and healthy fats helps regulate blood sugar levels and prevent the onset of type 2 diabetes. Reducing intake of refined sugars and processed foods is particularly important.
• **Cancer**: Antioxidant-rich foods, such as berries, leafy greens, and nuts, protect cells from oxidative damage and reduce cancer risk. Dietary fiber from whole plant foods supports a healthy digestive system and may lower the risk of colorectal cancer.

Immune Function and Inflammation

A healthy diet supports the immune system and helps reduce inflammation.

- **Immune Support**: Nutrients like vitamin C, vitamin D, zinc, and selenium play significant roles in immune function. These nutrients are abundant in fruits, vegetables, nuts, and seeds, making these foods vital for maintaining a robust immune system.

- **Anti-Inflammatory Foods**: Foods with anti-inflammatory properties, such as fatty fish, turmeric, and leafy greens, help manage and reduce chronic inflammation, which is a common underlying factor in diseases such as arthritis, heart disease, and Alzheimer's.

Mental Health and Cognitive Function

Nutrition significantly impacts mental health and cognitive function.

- **Brain Health**: Omega-3 fatty acids, found in fish and flaxseeds, are essential for brain health and cognitive function. These fats support neural development and help maintain mental acuity and memory.

- **Mood Regulation**: Nutrient-rich diets that include complex carbohydrates, lean proteins, and healthy fats support the production of neurotransmitters like serotonin and dopamine, which are crucial for mood regulation and mental well-being.

Weight Management and Energy Levels

Maintaining a healthy weight and stable energy levels are critical for overall health.

- **Weight Management**: A diet high in fiber, protein, and healthy fats helps control appetite and promote satiety, making it easier to maintain a healthy weight. Avoiding processed foods and sugary drinks is crucial in preventing weight gain and related health issues.

- **Energy Levels**: Consuming balanced meals that include a mix of macronutrients ensures sustained energy throughout the day. Hydration is also key, as water is vital for metabolic processes and maintaining energy levels.

A balanced, nutrient-rich diet supports the body's natural healing processes, prevents chronic diseases, boosts immune function, enhances mental health, and maintains healthy weight and energy levels. By adhering to dietary principles of consuming whole, natural foods and avoiding processed items, individuals can take proactive steps towards achieving lasting health and well-being.

Why Diet Matters

The link between diet and overall health is well-established. The foods we consume provide the necessary nutrients for the body to function correctly and maintain health.

- **_Disease Prevention_**: A nutritious diet helps prevent a range of chronic diseases, including heart disease, diabetes, and cancer. Foods rich in antioxidants, fiber, and healthy fats are particularly beneficial in reducing disease risk.

- **_Mental Health_**: Diet also plays a significant role in mental health. Nutrient-rich foods support brain function, improve mood, and reduce the risk of mental health disorders such as depression and anxiety. Omega-3 fatty acids, found in fish and flaxseeds, are essential for cognitive function.

- **_Energy Levels_**: Proper nutrition provides the energy needed for daily activities and overall vitality. Balanced meals that include a mix of macronutrients help maintain stable blood sugar levels and prevent fatigue.

How Nutrition Impacts the Body's Healing Processes

Nutrition directly influences the body's ability to heal and repair itself. Proper nutrients are essential for cellular repair, immune function, and inflammation control.

- **_Cellular Repair and Regeneration_**: Nutrients from a healthy diet are crucial for the repair and regeneration of cells. Proteins provide amino acids needed for new cell formation, while vitamins and minerals support various cellular functions.

- **_Immune Function_**: A strong immune system relies on a steady supply of nutrients. Vitamins C and D, zinc, and other micronutrients are vital for maintaining immune health and protecting against infections.

- **_Inflammation Control_**: Chronic inflammation can hinder the healing process. Anti-inflammatory foods, such as fatty fish, turmeric, and leafy greens, help manage and reduce inflammation, promoting better health and faster recovery.

Understanding why diet matters and how it impacts overall health and the body's healing processes can empower individuals to make informed dietary choices that support their long-term well-being.

By adhering to these principles, individuals can enhance their health, prevent chronic diseases, and support their body's natural healing abilities.

SELF-CARE PRACTICES: ENHANCING PHYSICAL AND MENTAL WELL-BEING

Beyond the nutritious and healing recipes, "The Anti-Inflammatory Diet" also places a strong emphasis on self-care routines and practices that complement a healthy diet. True wellness encompasses more than just what we eat; it includes how we care for our bodies and minds. This chapter provides you with practical tips and strategies to integrate self-care into your daily life, enhancing both your physical and mental well-being.

Daily Self-Care Practices

1. **Mindful Eating**

   o **Savor Each Bite:** Take the time to enjoy your meals without distractions. Focus on the flavors, textures, and aromas of your food.

   o **Listen to Your Body:** Pay attention to hunger and fullness cues. Eat when you're hungry and stop when you're satisfied.

   o **Chew Thoroughly:** Chewing your food thoroughly aids digestion and allows your body to better absorb nutrients.

2. **Hydration**

   o **Drink Plenty of Water:** Aim to drink at least 8 glasses of water a day. Proper hydration is crucial for all bodily functions.

   o **Herbal Teas and Infusions:** Incorporate herbal teas into your routine. They offer hydration and additional health benefits from herbs.

3. **Physical Activity**

   o **Move Regularly:** Incorporate physical activity into your daily routine. Whether it's a brisk walk, yoga, or a workout at the gym, regular exercise supports physical health and mental clarity.

   o **Stretching:** Begin and end your day with gentle stretching exercises to maintain flexibility and reduce muscle tension.

4. **Stress Management**

   o **Breathing Exercises:** Practice deep breathing exercises to calm the mind and reduce stress. Techniques such as diaphragmatic breathing can be very effective.

   o **Meditation and Mindfulness:** Set aside time each day for meditation or mindfulness practices. These can help center your thoughts and reduce anxiety.

5. **Sleep Hygiene**

   o **Establish a Routine:** Go to bed and wake up at the same time each day to regulate your body's internal clock.

- Create a Relaxing Environment: Make your bedroom a sanctuary for sleep. Keep it cool, dark, and quiet, and invest in a comfortable mattress and pillows.

- Limit Screen Time: Avoid screens at least an hour before bedtime to improve sleep quality.

6. **Nutrient-Rich Snacks**

- Healthy Snacks: Choose nutrient-dense snacks like fruits, nuts, and seeds. They provide sustained energy and essential nutrients without the crash associated with sugary snacks.

- Preparation: Keep healthy snacks readily available. Pre-cut veggies, portioned nuts, and easy-to-grab fruits can make choosing healthy options easier.

7. **Emotional Wellness**

- Journaling: Take a few minutes each day to write down your thoughts and feelings. Journaling can help process emotions and provide mental clarity.

- Connect with Loved Ones: Maintain social connections with friends and family. Social support is vital for emotional health.

Incorporating these self-care practices into your daily routine doesn't have to be overwhelming. Start by choosing one or two practices that resonate with you and gradually add more as you become comfortable. The goal is to create a sustainable self-care routine that enhances your well-being and fits seamlessly into your lifestyle.

BREAKFAST RECIPES

Green Goddess Smoothie Bowl

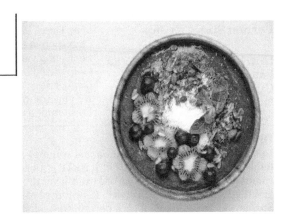

Prepping Time: 10 min.
Cooking Time: 0 min.
Portion Size: 1 bowl

Ingredients:
- 1 cup spinach leaves
- 1/2 avocado
- 1 banana
- 1/2 cup Greek yogurt
- 1 table spoon chia seeds
- 1/2 cup unsweetened almond milk
- 1 tablespoon honey (optional)
- 1 teaspoon spirulina powder

Toppings:
Fresh Berries
Sliced Kiwi
Sliced Almonds
Coconut flakes

Nutritional Data: 350 calories | 10g protein | 18g fat | 45g carbohydrates | 12g fiber | 20g sugar | 120mg sodium

Directions:
In a blender, combine spinach leaves, avocado, banana, Greek yogurt, almond milk, chia seeds, honey (if using), and spirulina powder. Blend until smooth and creamy. Pour the smoothie into a bowl. Top with fresh berries, sliced kiwi, sliced almonds, and coconut flakes. Serve immediately and enjoy your nutritious Green Goddess Smoothie Bowl.

Protein-Packed Overnight Chia Pudding

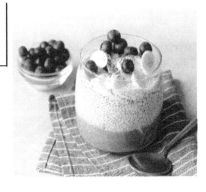

Prepping Time: 10 minutes
Cooking Time: 0 minutes (overnight refrigeration)
Portion Size: 2 servings

Nutritional Data: 300 calories
Protein: 12g | Fat: 14g
Carbohydrates: 34g | Fiber: 12g
Sugar: 15g | Sodium: 120mg

Ingredients:
1/2 cup chia seeds
2 cups unsweetened almond milk
1/2 cup Greek yogurt
2 tablespoons honey or maple syrup
1 teaspoon vanilla extract
Fresh fruits for topping (e.g., berries, banana slices)
Nuts and seeds for topping (e.g., almonds, sunflower seeds)

Directions:
In a medium-sized bowl, whisk together chia seeds, almond milk, Greek yogurt, honey or maple syrup, and vanilla extract until well combined. Cover the bowl and refrigerate overnight or for at least 4 hours, allowing the chia seeds to absorb the liquid and thicken. Stir the mixture before serving to ensure an even consistency. Divide the chia pudding into two portions. Top each serving with fresh fruits, nuts, and seeds of your choice.
Serve immediately and enjoy your nutritious and protein-packed overnight chia pudding.

Quinoa and Berry Breakfast Parfait

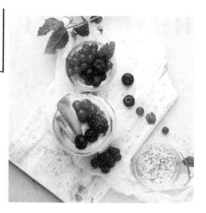

Prepping Time: 15 minutes
Cooking Time: 15 minutes
(overnight refrigeration)
Portion Size: 2 servings

Nutritional Data: 320 calories
Protein: 12g | Fat: 8g
Carbohydrates: 50g | Fiber: 6g
Sugar: 20g | Sodium: 50mg

Ingredients:
1/2 cup quinoa, rinsed
1 cup water
1 cup Greek yogurt
1 tablespoon honey or maple syrup
1 teaspoon vanilla extract
1 cup mixed berries (strawberries, blueberries, raspberries)
1/4 cup granola
Fresh mint leaves for garnish (optional)

Directions:
In a small saucepan, bring quinoa and water to a boil. Reduce heat to low, cover, and simmer for 15 minutes or until quinoa is tender and water is absorbed. Let it cool completely. In a bowl, mix Greek yogurt, honey or maple syrup, and vanilla extract until smooth. In two serving glasses or bowls, layer the ingredients starting with a layer of quinoa, followed by a layer of yogurt mixture, and then a layer of mixed berries. Repeat the layers until all ingredients are used, finishing with berries on top.
Sprinkle granola on top of each parfait. Garnish with fresh mint leaves if desired.
Serve immediately and enjoy your nutritious quinoa and berry breakfast parfait.

Spinach and Avocado Power Smoothie

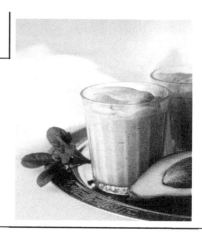

Prepping Time: 5 minutes
Cooking Time: 0 minutes
Portion Size: 1 smoothie

Nutritional Data: 280 calories
Protein: 5g | Fat: 18g
Carbohydrates: 32g | Fiber: 11g
Sugar: 12g | Sodium: 105 mg

Ingredients:
1 cup fresh spinach leaves
1/2 ripe avocado
1 banana
1 cup unsweetened almond milk
1 tablespoon chia seeds
1 teaspoon honey (optional)
Ice cubes (optional, for a thicker consistency)

Directions:
Combine spinach leaves, avocado, banana, almond milk, chia seeds, and honey (if using) in a blender.
Blend until smooth and creamy. Add ice cubes if a thicker consistency is desired and blend again.
Pour into a glass and serve immediately.

Hearty Buckwheat Porridge with Nuts and Seeds

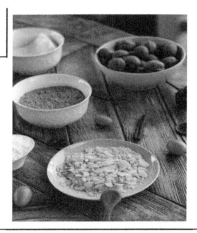

Prepping Time: 15 minutes
Cooking Time: 5 minutes
Portion Size: 2 servings

Nutritional Data: 350 calories
Protein: 10g | Fat: 14g
Carbohydrates: 45g | Fiber: 10g
Sugar: 12g | Sodium: 80mg

Ingredients:
1 cup buckwheat groats
2 cups water
1 cup almond milk
1 tablespoon honey or maple syrup
1 teaspoon cinnamon
1/4 cup chopped almonds
1/4 cup pumpkin seeds
1 tablespoon chia seeds
1 tablespoon flaxseeds
Fresh berries for topping (optional)

Directions:
Rinse buckwheat groats under cold water.
In a medium saucepan, bring water to a boil. Add buckwheat groats, reduce heat to low, cover, and simmer for about 10 minutes, or until the water is absorbed. Stir in almond milk, honey or maple syrup, and cinnamon. Continue to cook on low heat for another 5 minutes, stirring occasionally, until the porridge is creamy.
Divide the porridge into two bowls. Top with chopped almonds, pumpkin seeds, chia seeds, flaxseeds, and fresh berries if desired.
Serve immediately and enjoy your hearty and nutritious buckwheat porridge.

Veggie-Loaded Chickpea Breakfast Wrap

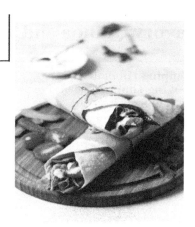

Prepping Time: 10 minutes
Cooking Time: 10 minutes
Portion Size: 2 wraps

Nutritional Data: 400 calories
Protein: 12g | Fat: 18g
Carbohydrates: 50g | Fiber: 12g
Sugar: 8g | Sodium: 600 mg

Ingredients:
1 cup canned chickpeas, drained and rinsed
1/2 cup diced bell pepper (any color)
1/2 cup diced tomatoes
1/4 cup chopped red onion
1/4 cup chopped fresh spinach
2 tablespoons olive oil
1 teaspoon ground cumin
1/2 teaspoon smoked paprika
Salt and pepper to taste
2 whole wheat or gluten-free wraps
1/4 cup hummus
Fresh cilantro or parsley for garnish (optional)

Directions:
Heat olive oil in a large skillet over medium heat. Add the red onion and bell pepper, sauté for 3-4 minutes until softened.
Add the chickpeas, tomatoes, cumin, smoked paprika, salt, and pepper. Cook for another 5-6 minutes, stirring occasionally, until the chickpeas are heated through and slightly crispy. Stir in the fresh spinach and cook for an additional 1-2 minutes until wilted.
Warm the wraps in a dry skillet or microwave. Spread a layer of hummus on each wrap. Divide the chickpea mixture between the two wraps, placing it in the center of each. Roll up the wraps, folding in the sides as you go.
Garnish with fresh cilantro or parsley if desired.
Serve immediately and enjoy your veggie-loaded chickpea breakfast wrap.

Blueberry Almond Overnight Oats

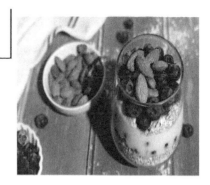

Prepping Time: 10 minutes
Cooking Time: 0 minutes
(overnight refrigeration)
Portion Size: 2 servings

Nutritional Data: 320 calories
Protein: 12g | Fat: 10g
Carbohydrates: 45g | Fiber: 8g
Sugar: 15g | Sodium: 85 mg

Ingredients:
1 cup rolled oats
1 cup unsweetened almond milk
1/2 cup Greek yogurt
2 tablespoons chia seeds
1 tablespoon honey or maple syrup
1 teaspoon vanilla extract
1 cup fresh blueberries
1/4 cup sliced almonds

Directions:
In a medium-sized bowl, combine rolled oats, almond milk, Greek yogurt, chia seeds, honey or maple syrup, and vanilla extract. Stir well to combine.
Gently fold in the fresh blueberries and sliced almonds.
Divide the mixture evenly between two jars or containers with lids.
Cover and refrigerate overnight, or for at least 4 hours.
In the morning, give the oats a good stir. Add a splash of almond milk if the mixture is too thick.
Serve cold, topped with additional blueberries and almonds if desired.

Savory Quinoa and Veggie Breakfast Bowl

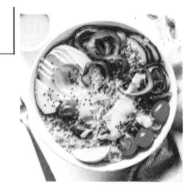

Prepping Time: 10 minutes
Cooking Time: 20 minutes
Portion Size: 2 servings

Nutritional Data: 400 calories
Protein: 12g | Fat: 18g
Carbohydrates: 50g | Fiber: 12g
Sugar: 8g | Sodium: 250 mg

Ingredients:
1 cup quinoa, rinsed
2 cups water
1 tablespoon olive oil
1/2 cup diced bell pepper
1/2 cup diced zucchini
1/2 cup cherry tomatoes, halved
1/4 cup red onion, finely chopped
2 cups fresh spinach leaves
2 tablespoons nutritional yeast
Salt and pepper to taste
1 avocado, sliced
Fresh parsley for garnish (optional)

Directions:
In a medium saucepan, bring water to a boil. Add the quinoa, reduce heat to low, cover, and simmer for about 15 minutes, or until the water is absorbed and the quinoa is tender. Fluff with a fork and set aside.
In a large skillet, heat the olive oil over medium heat. Add the red onion and sauté for 2-3 minutes until softened.
Add the bell pepper and zucchini, and cook for another 5 minutes until the vegetables are tender.
Stir in the cherry tomatoes and cook for an additional 2 minutes. Add the fresh spinach leaves and cook until wilted, about 1-2 minutes. Mix the cooked quinoa into the skillet with the vegetables. Stir in the nutritional yeast, and season with salt and pepper to taste. Divide the quinoa and veggie mixture between two bowls.
Top each bowl with sliced avocado and garnish with fresh parsley if desired.
Serve immediately and enjoy your savory quinoa and veggie breakfast bowl.

Coconut and Mango Chia Seed Pudding

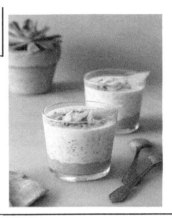

Prepping Time: 10 minutes
Cooking Time: 0 minutes
(overnight refrigeration)
Portion Size: 2 servings

Nutritional Data: 300 calories
Protein: 6g | Fat: 18g
Carbohydrates: 35g | Fiber: 12g
Sugar: 20g | Sodium: 90 mg

Ingredients:
1/2 cup chia seeds
1 cup coconut milk
1/2 cup unsweetened almond milk
1 tablespoon honey or maple syrup
1 teaspoon vanilla extract
1 cup fresh mango, diced
2 tablespoons unsweetened shredded coconut

Directions:
In a medium-sized bowl, whisk together chia seeds, coconut milk, almond milk, honey or maple syrup, and vanilla extract until well combined.
Cover the bowl and refrigerate overnight, or for at least 4 hours, allowing the chia seeds to absorb the liquid and thicken.
Stir the mixture before serving to ensure an even consistency.
Divide the chia pudding into two portions.
Top each serving with diced fresh mango and a sprinkle of shredded coconut.
Serve immediately and enjoy your refreshing coconut and mango chia seed pudding.

Kale and Sweet Potato Breakfast Hash

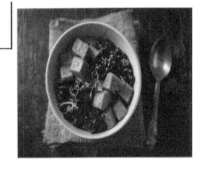

Prepping Time: 10 minutes
Cooking Time: 20 minutes
Portion Size: 2 servings

Nutritional Data: 350 calories
Protein: 8g | Fat: 18g
Carbohydrates: 40g | Fiber: 8g
Sugar: 10g | Sodium: 320 mg

Ingredients:
2 tablespoons olive oil
1 medium sweet potato, peeled and diced
1 small red onion, diced
1 red bell pepper, diced
2 cups fresh kale, chopped
2 garlic cloves, minced
1/2 teaspoon smoked paprika
Salt and pepper to taste
2 eggs (optional, for serving)
Fresh parsley for garnish (optional)

Directions:
Heat olive oil in a large skillet over medium heat.
Add the diced sweet potato and cook for about 10 minutes, stirring occasionally, until they begin to soften.
Add the red onion and red bell pepper to the skillet. Cook for another 5 minutes until the vegetables are tender.
Stir in the garlic, smoked paprika, salt, and pepper. Cook for 1-2 minutes until fragrant.
Add the chopped kale and cook until wilted, about 2-3 minutes.
If using eggs, create small wells in the hash and crack an egg into each well. Cover the skillet and cook until the eggs are set to your liking. Garnish with fresh parsley if desired.
Serve immediately and enjoy your nutritious kale and sweet potato breakfast hash.

Tropical Green Smoothie with Spirulina

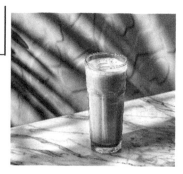

Prepping Time: 5 minutes
Cooking Time: 0 minutes
Portion Size: 1 smoothie

Nutritional Data: 250 calories
Protein: 4g | Fat: 2g
Carbohydrates: 60g | Fiber: 6g
Sugar: 35g | Sodium: 60 mg

Ingredients:
1 cup fresh spinach leaves
1/2 cup frozen mango chunks
1/2 cup frozen pineapple chunks
1 banana
1 cup coconut water
1 teaspoon spirulina powder
Juice of 1 lime
Ice cubes (optional, for thicker consistency)

Directions:
Combine spinach leaves, mango chunks, pineapple chunks, banana, coconut water, spirulina powder, and lime juice in a blender.
Blend until smooth and creamy. Add ice cubes if a thicker consistency is desired and blend again.
Pour into a glass and serve immediately.

Apple Cinnamon Quinoa Breakfast Bake

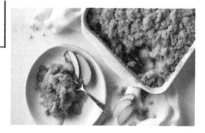

Prepping Time: 15 minutes
Cooking Time: 40 minutes
Portion Size: 4 servings

Nutritional Data: 300 calories
Protein: 8g | Fat: 8g
Carbohydrates: 54g | Fiber: 6g
Sugar: 20g | Sodium: 200 mg

Ingredients:
1 cup quinoa, rinsed
2 large apples, peeled, cored, and diced
1 cup unsweetened almond milk
1/2 cup water
1/4 cup maple syrup
1 teaspoon vanilla extract
1 teaspoon ground cinnamon
1/2 teaspoon ground nutmeg
1/4 teaspoon salt
1/4 cup chopped walnuts (optional)
1/4 cup raisins (optional)

Directions:
Preheat the oven to 350°F (175°C) and lightly grease an 8x8-inch baking dish.
In a medium saucepan, combine quinoa, almond milk, water, maple syrup, vanilla extract, cinnamon, nutmeg, and salt. Bring to a boil over medium heat.
Reduce heat to low, cover, and simmer for about 15 minutes, or until the quinoa is tender and most of the liquid is absorbed.
Stir in the diced apples, chopped walnuts, and raisins.
Pour the quinoa mixture into the prepared baking dish and spread evenly.
Bake for 20-25 minutes, or until the top is golden brown and the apples are tender.
Let cool for a few minutes before serving.

Zucchini and Carrot Breakfast Muffins

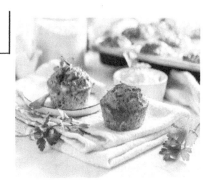

Prepping Time: 15 minutes
Cooking Time: 25 minutes
Portion Size: 12 muffins

Nutritional Data: 180 calories
Protein: 4g | Fat: 8g
Carbohydrates: 24g | Fiber: 3g
Sugar: 10g | Sodium: 180 mg

Ingredients:
1 cup grated zucchini
1 cup grated carrot
2 cups whole wheat flour
1/2 cup rolled oats
1/2 cup honey or maple syrup
1/2 cup unsweetened applesauce
1/4 cup coconut oil, melted
2 large eggs
1 teaspoon vanilla extract
1 teaspoon baking soda
1 teaspoon ground cinnamon
1/2 teaspoon ground nutmeg
1/2 teaspoon salt
1/2 cup chopped walnuts (optional)
1/4 cup raisins (optional)

Directions:
Preheat the oven to 350°F (175°C) and line a 12-cup muffin tin with paper liners or lightly grease it.
In a large bowl, whisk together the flour, rolled oats, baking soda, cinnamon, nutmeg, and salt.
In another bowl, beat the eggs and then mix in the honey or maple syrup, applesauce, coconut oil, and vanilla extract.
Add the wet ingredients to the dry ingredients and stir until just combined.
Fold in the grated zucchini, grated carrot, walnuts, and raisins.
Divide the batter evenly among the 12 muffin cups. Bake for 20-25 minutes, or until a toothpick inserted into the center of a muffin comes out clean.
Allow the muffins to cool in the tin for 5 minutes before transferring to a wire rack to cool completely.

Banana Walnut Overnight Oats

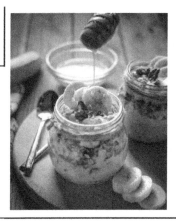

Prepping Time: 10 minutes
Cooking Time: 0 minutes
(overnight refrigeration)
Portion Size: 2 servings

Nutritional Data: 320 calories
Protein: 10g | Fat: 12g
Carbohydrates: 45g | Fiber: 7g
Sugar: 15g | Sodium: 70 mg

Ingredients:
1 cup rolled oats
1 cup unsweetened almond milk
1/2 cup Greek yogurt
1 banana, mashed
2 tablespoons honey or maple syrup
1 teaspoon vanilla extract
1/2 teaspoon ground cinnamon
1/4 cup chopped walnuts
Banana slices and extra walnuts for topping (optional)

Directions:
In a medium-sized bowl, combine rolled oats, almond milk, Greek yogurt, mashed banana, honey or maple syrup, vanilla extract, and ground cinnamon. Stir well to combine.
Fold in the chopped walnuts.
Divide the mixture evenly between two jars or containers with lids.
Cover and refrigerate overnight, or for at least 4 hours.
In the morning, give the oats a good stir. Add a splash of almond milk if the mixture is too thick.
Serve cold, topped with banana slices and extra walnuts if desired.

Berry Blast Smoothie with Chia Seeds

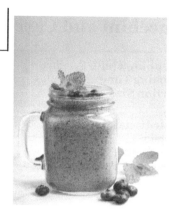

Prepping Time: 5 minutes
Cooking Time: 0 minutes
Portion Size: 1 smoothie

Nutritional Data: 220 calories
Protein: 5g | Fat: 4g
Carbohydrates: 45g | Fiber: 10g
Sugar: 25g | Sodium: 80 mg

Ingredients:
1 cup mixed berries (blueberries, strawberries, raspberries)
1 banana
1 cup unsweetened almond milk
1 tablespoon chia seeds
1 tablespoon honey or maple syrup (optional)
1/2 cup Greek yogurt (optional for added creaminess)
Ice cubes (optional, for a thicker consistency)

Directions:
Combine mixed berries, banana, almond milk, chia seeds, honey or maple syrup (if using), and Greek yogurt (if using) in a blender.
Blend until smooth and creamy. Add ice cubes if a thicker consistency is desired and blend again.
Pour into a glass and serve immediately.

Herbed Avocado and Tomato Breakfast Toast

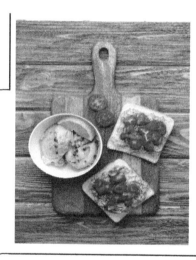

Prepping Time: 10 minutes
Cooking Time: 0 minutes
Portion Size: 2 servings

Nutritional Data: 300 calories
Protein: 5g | Fat: 20g
Carbohydrates: 28g | Fiber: 8g
Sugar: 4g | Sodium: 350 mg

Ingredients:
2 slices whole-grain bread, toasted
1 ripe avocado
1 cup cherry tomatoes, halved
1 tablespoon fresh lemon juice
1 tablespoon olive oil
1/4 teaspoon sea salt
1/4 teaspoon black pepper
1 tablespoon chopped fresh basil
1 tablespoon chopped fresh parsley
1 tablespoon chopped fresh chives

Directions:
In a small bowl, mash the avocado with a fork. Stir in the lemon juice, sea salt, and black pepper until well combined.
In another bowl, toss the cherry tomatoes with olive oil and a pinch of sea salt.
Spread the mashed avocado mixture evenly onto the toasted bread slices.
Top with the halved cherry tomatoes.
Sprinkle chopped fresh basil, parsley, and chives over the tomatoes.
Serve immediately and enjoy your flavorful herbed avocado and tomato breakfast toast.

Pumpkin Spice Chia Pudding

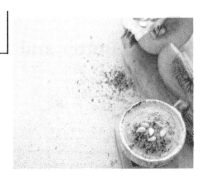

Prepping Time: 10 minutes
Cooking Time: 0 minutes
(overnight refrigeration)
Portion Size: 2 servings

Nutritional Data: 250 calories
Protein: 6g | Fat: 10g
Carbohydrates: 34g | Fiber: 14g
Sugar: 12g | Sodium: 100 mg

Ingredients:
1/2 cup chia seeds
1 cup unsweetened almond milk
1/2 cup pumpkin puree
2 tablespoons maple syrup
1 teaspoon vanilla extract
1 teaspoon ground cinnamon
1/2 teaspoon ground nutmeg
1/4 teaspoon ground ginger
1/4 teaspoon ground cloves

Directions:
In a medium-sized bowl, whisk together almond milk, pumpkin puree, maple syrup, vanilla extract, ground cinnamon, ground nutmeg, ground ginger, and ground cloves until well combined.
Stir in the chia seeds. Cover the bowl and refrigerate overnight, or for at least 4 hours, allowing the chia seeds to absorb the liquid and thicken. Stir the mixture before serving to ensure an even consistency.
Divide the chia pudding into two portions.
Serve cold, and enjoy your pumpkin spice chia pudding.

Smashed Chickpea and Avocado

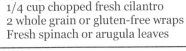

Prepping Time: 10 minutes
Cooking Time: 0 minutes
Portion Size: 2 slices of bread

Nutritional Data: 380 calories
Protein: 10g | Fat: 18g
Carbohydrates: 45g | Fiber: 12g
Sugar: 5g | Sodium: 400 mg

Ingredients:
1 can (15 oz) chickpeas, drained and rinsed
1 ripe avocado
1 tablespoon fresh lemon juice
1 tablespoon olive oil
1/4 teaspoon sea salt
1/4 teaspoon black pepper
1/2 teaspoon cumin
1/2 teaspoon smoked paprika
1/4 cup chopped red onion
1/4 cup chopped fresh cilantro
2 whole grain or gluten-free wraps
Fresh spinach or arugula leaves

Directions:
Mashed chickpeas and avocado
In a medium-sized bowl, mash the chickpeas and avocado until well combined but still chunky.
Add the lemon juice, olive oil, sea salt, black pepper, cumin, and smoked paprika.
Add chopped red onion and fresh cilantro.
Spread on two slices of whole wheat bread and spread an even amount of the chickpea and avocado mixture on each.
Top with fresh spinach leaves or arugula.
Serve immediately and enjoy your chickpeas and avocado.

Almond Butter and Banana Breakfast Bowl

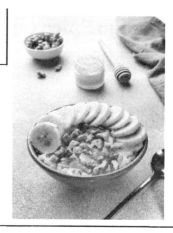

Prepping Time: 10 minutes
Cooking Time: 0 minutes
Portion Size: 1 bowl

Nutritional Data: 400 calories
Protein: 18g | Fat: 18g
Carbohydrates: 45g | Fiber: 8g
Sugar: 20g | Sodium: 125 mg

Ingredients:
1 cup plain Greek yogurt
1 banana, sliced
2 tablespoons almond butter
1 tablespoon chia seeds
1/4 cup granola
1 tablespoon honey (optional)
1/4 teaspoon ground cinnamon

Directions:
In a bowl, spoon the Greek yogurt as the base.
Top with sliced banana, almond butter, chia seeds, and granola.
Drizzle with honey if desired and sprinkle with ground cinnamon.
Serve immediately and enjoy your delicious and nutritious breakfast bowl.

Superfood Acai Bowl with Fresh Berries

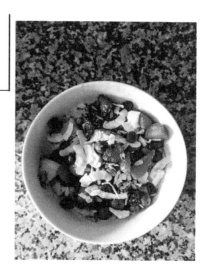

Prepping Time: 10 minutes
Cooking Time: 0 minutes
Portion Size: 1 bowl

Nutritional Data: 350 calories
Protein: 6g | Fat: 12g
Carbohydrates: 55g | Fiber: 14g
Sugar: 25g | Sodium: 80 mg

Ingredients:
1 packet frozen acai puree (100 grams)
1/2 banana
1/2 cup frozen mixed berries
1/2 cup unsweetened almond milk
1 tablespoon chia seeds
1 tablespoon honey or maple syrup (optional)

Toppings:
1/4 cup fresh blueberries
1/4 cup fresh strawberries, sliced
1/4 cup granola
1 tablespoon shredded coconut
1 tablespoon pumpkin seeds
Fresh mint leaves for garnish (optional)

Directions:
In a blender, combine the acai puree, banana, frozen mixed berries, almond milk, chia seeds, and honey or maple syrup (if using).
Blend until smooth and creamy. Pour the mixture into a bowl.
Top with fresh blueberries, strawberries, granola, shredded coconut, and pumpkin seeds.
Garnish with fresh mint leaves if desired.
Serve immediately and enjoy your nutrient-packed superfood acai bowl.

LUNCH RECIPES

Quinoa & Kale Salad with Lemon-Tahini Dressing

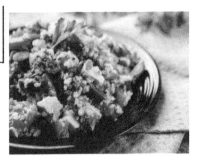

Prepping Time: 15 minutes
Cooking Time: 15 minutes
Portion Size: 4 servings

Nutritional Data: 400 calories
Protein: 12g | Fat: 18g
Carbohydrates: 48g | Fiber: 8g
Sugar: 10g | Sodium: 200 mg

Ingredients:
For the Salad:

1 cup quinoa, rinsed
2 cups water
4 cups chopped kale, stems removed
1 cup cherry tomatoes, halved
1/2 cup shredded carrots
1/4 cup chopped red onion
1/4 cup sunflower seeds
1/4 cup dried cranberries
For the Lemon-Tahini Dressing:
1/4 cup tahini
1/4 cup fresh lemon juice
2 tablespoons olive oil
1 tablespoon maple syrup
1 garlic clove, minced
1/4 teaspoon sea salt
1/4 teaspoon black pepper
2-3 tablespoons water (to thin, if needed)

Directions:
In a medium saucepan, bring the quinoa and water to a boil. Reduce the heat to low, cover, and simmer for about 15 minutes, or until the water is absorbed and the quinoa is tender. Let it cool. In a large bowl, combine the chopped kale, cherry tomatoes, shredded carrots, chopped red onion, sunflower seeds, and dried cranberries. In a small bowl, whisk together tahini, fresh lemon juice, olive oil, maple syrup, minced garlic, sea salt, and black pepper. Add water as needed to achieve a smooth, pourable consistency. Add the cooled quinoa to the salad bowl and toss to combine. Pour the lemon-tahini dressing over the salad and toss to coat evenly. Serve immediately or refrigerate for later.

Chickpea and Avocado Stuffed Bell Peppers

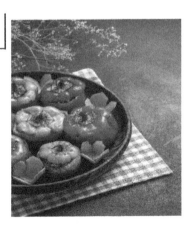

Prepping Time: 15 minutes
Cooking Time: 0 minutes
Portion Size: 4 servings

Nutritional Data: 280 calories
Protein: 7g | Fat: 14g
Carbohydrates: 34g | Fiber: 10g
Sugar: 5g | Sodium: 220 mg

Ingredients:
4 large bell peppers (any color), halved and seeds removed
1 can (15 oz) chickpeas, drained and rinsed
2 ripe avocados, diced
1/2 cup cherry tomatoes, halved
1/4 cup red onion, finely chopped
1/4 cup fresh cilantro, chopped
2 tablespoons fresh lime juice
1 tablespoon olive oil
1/2 teaspoon sea salt
1/4 teaspoon black pepper
1/2 teaspoon cumin
1/2 teaspoon smoked paprika

Directions:
In a large bowl, mash the chickpeas with a fork until they are mostly broken down but still have some texture. Add the diced avocados, cherry tomatoes, red onion, fresh cilantro, lime juice, olive oil, sea salt, black pepper, cumin, and smoked paprika. Stir gently to combine. Spoon the chickpea and avocado mixture into the halved bell peppers, filling each half generously. Arrange the stuffed bell peppers on a serving platter. Serve immediately and enjoy your dish.

Grilled Vegetable and Hummus Wrap

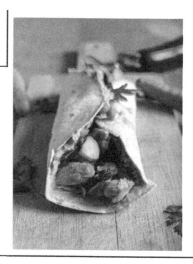

Prepping Time: 10 minutes
Cooking Time: 15 minutes
Portion Size: 2 wraps

Nutritional Data: 320 calories
Protein: 8g | Fat: 14g
Carbohydrates: 40g | Fiber: 8g
Sugar: 6g | Sodium: 350 mg

Ingredients:
1 small zucchini, sliced
1 small eggplant, sliced
1 red bell pepper, sliced
1 yellow bell pepper, sliced
1 tablespoon olive oil
Salt and pepper to taste
1/2 teaspoon dried oregano
1/2 teaspoon dried thyme
1/2 cup hummus
2 whole grain or gluten-free wraps
1 cup fresh spinach leaves

Directions:
Preheat the grill to medium-high heat.
In a bowl, toss the zucchini, eggplant, and bell peppers with olive oil, salt, pepper, oregano, and thyme until evenly coated.
Grill the vegetables for about 5-7 minutes on each side, until tender and slightly charred.
Remove the vegetables from the grill and set aside to cool slightly. Spread 1/4 cup of hummus onto each wrap.
Arrange the grilled vegetables and fresh spinach leaves evenly on top of the hummus. Roll up the wraps, folding in the sides as you go. Slice the wraps in half and serve immediately.

Lentil and Spinach Soup with Turmeric

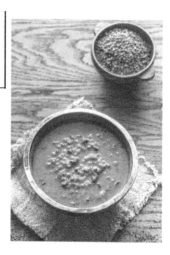

Prepping Time: 10 minutes
Cooking Time: 30 minutes
Portion Size: 4 servings

Nutritional Data: 230 calories
Protein: 12g | Fat: 5g
Carbohydrates: 34g | Fiber: 12g
Sugar: 4g | Sodium: 450 mg

Ingredients:
1 tablespoon olive oil
1 medium onion, chopped
2 garlic cloves, minced
1 cup dried red lentils, rinsed
1 teaspoon ground turmeric
1 teaspoon ground cumin
1/2 teaspoon ground coriander
1/2 teaspoon ground ginger
6 cups vegetable broth
2 cups fresh spinach leaves, chopped
1 medium carrot, diced
1 celery stalk, diced
Salt and pepper to taste
Juice of 1 lemon
Fresh cilantro for garnish (optional)

Directions:
In a large pot, heat the olive oil over medium heat. Add the chopped onion and garlic, and sauté until softened, about 5 minutes.
Stir in the lentils, turmeric, cumin, coriander, and ginger, and cook for another minute until fragrant.
Add the vegetable broth, carrot, and celery. Bring to a boil, then reduce heat and simmer for about 20 minutes, or until the lentils and vegetables are tender. Stir in the chopped spinach and cook for an additional 5 minutes until wilted.
Season with salt, pepper, and lemon juice to taste.
Serve hot, garnished with fresh cilantro if desired.

Rainbow Veggie Buddha Bowl

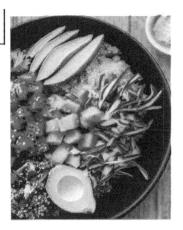

Prepping Time: 15 minutes
Cooking Time: 20 minutes
Portion Size: 2 bowls

Nutritional Data: 450 calories
Protein: 12g | Fat: 22g
Carbohydrates: 52g | Fiber: 12g
Sugar: 10g | Sodium: 300 mg

Ingredients:
1 cup quinoa, rinsed
2 cups water
1 cup cherry tomatoes, halved
1 cup shredded red cabbage
1 cup sliced cucumbers
1 cup shredded carrots
1 avocado, sliced
1 cup chickpeas, drained and rinsed
2 tablespoons olive oil
1 tablespoon lemon juice
1 teaspoon ground cumin
Salt and pepper to taste
Fresh cilantro for garnish (optional)
Tahini Dressing:
1/4 cup tahini
2 tablespoons fresh lemon juice
1 tablespoon maple syrup
1 garlic clove, minced
2-3 tablespoons water (to thin)
Salt and pepper to taste

Directions:
In a medium saucepan, bring the quinoa and water to a boil. Reduce heat to low, cover, and simmer for about 15 minutes, or until the quinoa is tender and the water is absorbed. Let it cool slightly. In a bowl, toss the chickpeas with olive oil, lemon juice, ground cumin, salt, and pepper. In a small bowl, whisk together tahini, lemon juice, maple syrup, minced garlic, and water until smooth. Season with salt and pepper to taste. Divide the cooked quinoa between two bowls. Arrange the cherry tomatoes, red cabbage, cucumbers, shredded carrots, avocado slices, and chickpeas on top of the quinoa. Drizzle the tahini dressing over the bowls. Garnish with fresh cilantro if desired
Serve immediately and enjoy your colorful and nutritious Rainbow Veggie Buddha Bowl.

Lentil and Spinach Soup with Turmeric

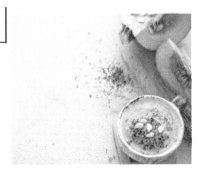

Prepping Time: 10 minutes
Cooking Time: 30 minutes
Portion Size: 4 servings

Nutritional Data: 230 calories
Protein: 12g | Fat: 5g
Carbohydrates: 34g | Fiber: 12g
Sugar: 4g | Sodium: 450 mg

Ingredients:
1 tablespoon olive oil
1 medium onion, chopped
2 garlic cloves, minced
1 cup dried red lentils, rinsed
1 teaspoon ground turmeric
1 teaspoon ground cumin
1/2 teaspoon ground coriander
1/2 teaspoon ground ginger
6 cups vegetable broth
2 cups fresh spinach leaves, chopped
1 medium carrot, diced
1 celery stalk, diced
Salt and pepper to taste
Juice of 1 lemon
Fresh cilantro for garnish (optional)

Directions:
In a large pot, heat the olive oil over medium heat. Add the chopped onion and garlic, and sauté until softened, about 5 minutes. Stir in the lentils, turmeric, cumin, coriander, and ginger, and cook for another minute until fragrant.
Add the vegetable broth, carrot, and celery. Bring to a boil, then reduce heat and simmer for about 20 minutes, or until the lentils and vegetables are tender. Stir in the chopped spinach and cook for an additional 5 minutes until wilted.
Season with salt, pepper, and lemon juice to taste. Serve hot, garnished with fresh cilantro if desired.

Spaghetti Squash with Pesto and Cherry Tomatoes

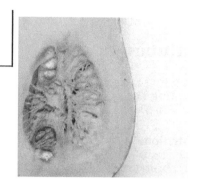

Prepping Time: 10 minutes
Cooking Time: 40 minutes
Portion Size: 4 servings

Nutritional Data: 320 calories
Protein: 7g | Fat: 28g
Carbohydrates: 18g | Fiber: 4g
Sugar: 5g | Sodium: 180 mg

Ingredients:
1 large spaghetti squash
2 tablespoons olive oil
Salt and pepper to taste
1 cup cherry tomatoes, halved
1/4 cup fresh basil leaves, chopped
1/4 cup grated Parmesan cheese (optional)
1/4 cup pine nuts (optional)

For the Pesto:
2 cups fresh basil leaves
1/4 cup pine nuts
1/2 cup grated Parmesan cheese
2 garlic cloves
1/2 cup olive oil
Salt and pepper to taste

Directions:
Preheat the oven to 400°F (200°C). Cut the spaghetti squash in half lengthwise and scoop out the seeds. Drizzle the cut sides with olive oil and season with salt and pepper. Place the squash halves cut-side down on a baking sheet and roast for about 35-40 minutes, or until the flesh is tender and can be easily shredded with a fork.
While the squash is roasting, prepare the pesto. In a food processor, combine the basil leaves, pine nuts, Parmesan cheese, and garlic. Pulse until finely chopped. With the processor running, slowly add the olive oil until the mixture is smooth and creamy. Season with salt and pepper to taste. Once the squash is cooked, use a fork to scrape out the flesh into spaghetti-like strands and transfer to a large bowl. Add the cherry tomatoes, chopped basil, and pine nuts to the bowl with the spaghetti squash. Toss with the prepared pesto until well combined. Serve the spaghetti squash topped with additional grated Parmesan cheese if desired.

Mixed Bean Salad with Fresh Herbs

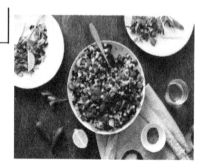

Prepping Time: 15 minutes
Cooking Time: 0 minutes
Portion Size: 4 servings

Nutritional Data: 320 calories
Protein: 12g | Fat: 14g
Carbohydrates: 36g | Fiber: 12g
Sugar: 5g | Sodium: 400 mg

Ingredients:
1 can (15 oz) black beans, drained and rinsed
1 can (15 oz) chickpeas, drained and rinsed
1 can (15 oz) kidney beans, drained and rinsed
1 cup cherry tomatoes, halved
1/2 red onion, finely chopped
1 cucumber, diced
1/4 cup fresh parsley, chopped
1/4 cup fresh cilantro, chopped
1/4 cup fresh mint, chopped

For the Dressing:
1/4 cup olive oil
2 tablespoons fresh lemon juice
1 tablespoon red wine vinegar
1 garlic clove, minced
1 teaspoon Dijon mustard
Salt and pepper to taste

Directions:
In a large bowl, combine the black beans, chickpeas, kidney beans, cherry tomatoes, red onion, cucumber, parsley, cilantro, and mint. In a small bowl, whisk together the olive oil, lemon juice, red wine vinegar, minced garlic, Dijon mustard, salt, and pepper until well combined. Pour the dressing over the bean and vegetable mixture and toss to coat evenly.
Serve immediately or refrigerate for up to 2 hours to allow the flavors to meld.

Sweet Potato and Black Bean Burrito Bowl

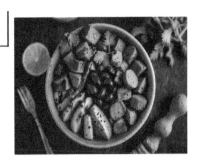

Prepping Time: 15 minutes
Cooking Time: 30 minutes
Portion Size: 4 servings

Nutritional Data: 420 calories
Protein: 12g | Fat: 15g
Carbohydrates: 58g | Fiber: 14g
Sugar: 8g | Sodium: 520 mg

Ingredients:
2 large sweet potatoes, peeled and diced
2 tablespoons olive oil
1 teaspoon ground cumin
1 teaspoon chili powder
Salt and pepper to taste
1 can (15 oz) black beans, drained and rinsed
1 cup cooked brown rice
1 cup cherry tomatoes, halved
1/2 red onion, finely chopped
1 avocado, diced
1/4 cup fresh cilantro, chopped
1 lime, cut into wedges

For the Dressing:
1/4 cup Greek yogurt
1 tablespoon fresh lime juice
1/2 teaspoon ground cumin
Salt and pepper to taste

Directions:
Preheat the oven to 400°F (200°C). In a large bowl, toss the diced sweet potatoes with olive oil, ground cumin, chili powder, salt, and pepper. Spread the sweet potatoes on a baking sheet and roast for 25-30 minutes, or until tender and slightly crispy.
In a small bowl, whisk together the Greek yogurt, lime juice, ground cumin, salt, and pepper to make the dressing. Set aside.
In a large bowl, combine the black beans, cooked brown rice, cherry tomatoes, red onion, avocado, and roasted sweet potatoes.
Drizzle the dressing over the bowl and toss to combine.
Garnish with fresh cilantro and serve with lime wedges on the side.

Zucchini Noodles with Avocado Basil Pesto

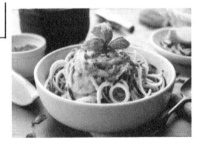

Prepping Time: 15 minutes
Cooking Time: 0 minutes
Portion Size: 2 servings

Nutritional Data: 350 calories
Protein: 8g | Fat: 30g
Carbohydrates: 16g | Fiber: 7g
Sugar: 6g | Sodium: 120 mg

Ingredients:
4 medium zucchinis, spiralized into noodles
1 ripe avocado
1 cup fresh basil leaves
1/4 cup pine nuts
1/4 cup grated Parmesan cheese
2 garlic cloves
2 tablespoons lemon juice
1/4 cup olive oil
Salt and pepper to taste
Cherry tomatoes for garnish (optional)

Directions:
In a food processor, combine the avocado, basil leaves, pine nuts, Parmesan cheese, garlic cloves, and lemon juice. Pulse until finely chopped. With the processor running, slowly add the olive oil until the mixture is smooth and creamy. Season with salt and pepper to taste. In a large bowl, toss the spiralized zucchini noodles with the avocado basil pesto until well coated.
Divide the zucchini noodles between two plates and garnish with cherry tomatoes if desired.
Serve immediately and enjoy your fresh and nutritious zucchini noodles with avocado basil pesto.

Cauliflower Rice Stir-Fry with Tofu

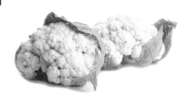

Prepping Time: 15 minutes
Cooking Time: 15 minutes
Portion Size: 4 servings

Nutritional Data: 250 calories
Protein: 15g | Fat: 12g
Carbohydrates: 20g | Fiber: 6g
Sugar: 6g | Sodium: 450 mg

Ingredients:
1 block (14 oz) firm tofu, drained and cubed
1 medium head of cauliflower, grated into rice-sized pieces
2 tablespoons sesame oil
1 red bell pepper, diced
1 cup snap peas, trimmed
1 cup shredded carrots
3 green onions, chopped
2 garlic cloves, minced
1 tablespoon grated fresh ginger
1/4 cup low-sodium soy sauce or tamari
2 tablespoons rice vinegar
1 tablespoon hoisin sauce (optional)
1 tablespoon sesame seeds (optional, for garnish)

Directions:
In a large skillet or wok, heat 1 tablespoon of sesame oil over medium-high heat. Add the cubed tofu and cook until golden brown on all sides, about 5-7 minutes. Remove the tofu from the skillet and set aside.
In the same skillet, add the remaining 1 tablespoon of sesame oil. Add the garlic and ginger and sauté for about 1 minute until fragrant. Add the red bell pepper, snap peas, and shredded carrots. Stir-fry for about 3-4 minutes until the vegetables are tender-crisp. Add the grated cauliflower rice and stir-fry for another 3-4 minutes until the cauliflower is tender.
Stir in the soy sauce, rice vinegar, and hoisin sauce (if using). Return the tofu to the skillet and toss to combine.
Garnish with sesame seeds and fresh cilantro if desired.
Serve immediately and enjoy your nutritious cauliflower rice stir-fry with tofu.

Hearty Minestrone Soup with Quinoa

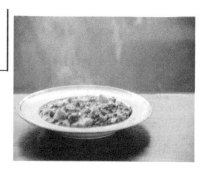

Prepping Time: 15 minutes
Cooking Time: 45 minutes
Portion Size: 6 servings

Nutritional Data: 230 calories
Protein: 8g | Fat: 5g
Carbohydrates: 38g | Fiber: 8g
Sugar: 6g | Sodium: 600 mg

Ingredients:
1 tablespoon olive oil
1 medium onion, chopped
2 garlic cloves, minced
2 carrots, diced
2 celery stalks, diced
1 zucchini, diced
1 yellow squash, diced
1 cup green beans, trimmed and cut into 1-inch pieces
1 can (15 oz) diced tomatoes
6 cups vegetable broth
1 can (15 oz) cannellini beans, drained and rinsed
1 cup cooked quinoa
1 teaspoon dried oregano
1 teaspoon dried basil
1/2 teaspoon dried thyme
Salt and pepper to taste
2 cups fresh spinach, chopped
1/4 cup fresh parsley, chopped (optional)
Grated Parmesan cheese for serving (optional)

Directions:
In a large pot, heat the olive oil over medium heat. Add the onion and garlic, and sauté until the onion is translucent, about 5 minutes. Add the carrots and celery, and cook for another 5 minutes until they begin to soften. Stir in the zucchini, yellow squash, and green beans, and cook for an additional 5 minutes. Add the diced tomatoes, vegetable broth, cannellini beans, cooked quinoa, oregano, basil, thyme, salt, and pepper. Bring the mixture to a boil, then reduce the heat and simmer for 25-30 minutes. Stir in the fresh spinach and cook until wilted, about 2 minutes. Serve hot, garnished with fresh parsley and grated Parmesan cheese if desired.

Stuffed Portobello Mushrooms with Spinach and Feta

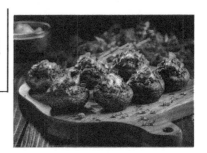

Prepping Time: 10 minutes
Cooking Time: 20 minutes
Portion Size: 4 servings

Nutritional Data: 180 calories
Protein: 7g | Fat: 12g
Carbohydrates: 12g | Fiber: 4g
Sugar: 3g | Sodium: 320 mg

Ingredients:
4 large portobello mushrooms, stems removed
2 tablespoons olive oil
1 small onion, finely chopped
2 garlic cloves, minced
4 cups fresh spinach leaves
1/2 cup crumbled feta cheese
1/4 cup breadcrumbs (optional)
Salt and pepper to taste
Fresh parsley for garnish (optional)

Directions:
Preheat the oven to 375°F (190°C). Brush the portobello mushrooms with 1 tablespoon of olive oil and place them on a baking sheet, gill side up. In a skillet, heat the remaining tablespoon of olive oil over medium heat. Add the chopped onion and garlic, and sauté until the onion is translucent, about 5 minutes.
Add the spinach to the skillet and cook until wilted, about 2-3 minutes. Season with salt and pepper to taste.
Remove the skillet from the heat and stir in the crumbled feta cheese and breadcrumbs if using.
Spoon the spinach and feta mixture evenly into each portobello mushroom cap.
Bake in the preheated oven for 15-20 minutes, or until the mushrooms are tender and the filling is heated through.
Garnish with fresh parsley if desired.
Serve immediately and enjoy your nutritious stuffed portobello mushrooms.

Greek Salad with Quinoa and Chickpeas

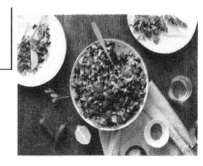

Prepping Time: 15 minutes
Cooking Time: 15 minutes
Portion Size: 4 servings

Nutritional Data: 360 calories
Protein: 12g | Fat: 18g
Carbohydrates: 40g | Fiber: 8g
Sugar: 5g | Sodium: 450 mg

Ingredients:
1 cup quinoa, rinsed
2 cups water
1 can (15 oz) chickpeas, drained and rinsed
1 cucumber, diced
1 cup cherry tomatoes, halved
1/2 red onion, finely chopped
1/2 cup Kalamata olives, pitted and halved
1/2 cup feta cheese, crumbled
1/4 cup fresh parsley, chopped

For the Dressing:
1/4 cup olive oil
2 tablespoons red wine vinegar
1 garlic clove, minced
1 teaspoon dried oregano
Salt and pepper to taste

Directions:
In a medium saucepan, bring the quinoa and water to a boil. Reduce heat to low, cover, and simmer for about 15 minutes, or until the quinoa is tender and the water is absorbed. Let it cool.
In a large bowl, combine the cooked quinoa, chickpeas, cucumber, cherry tomatoes, red onion, Kalamata olives, feta cheese, and fresh parsley. In a small bowl, whisk together the olive oil, red wine vinegar, minced garlic, dried oregano, salt, and pepper until well combined. Pour the dressing over the salad and toss to coat evenly.
Serve immediately or refrigerate for up to 2 hours to allow the flavors to meld.

Butternut Squash and Lentil Stew

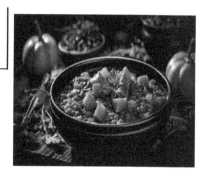

Prepping Time: 15 minutes
Cooking Time: 45 minutes
Portion Size: 4 servings

Nutritional Data: 320 calories
Protein: 12g | Fat: 8g
Carbohydrates: 52g | Fiber: 14g
Sugar: 9g | Sodium: 520 mg

Ingredients:
2 tablespoons olive oil
1 large onion, chopped
2 garlic cloves, minced
1 medium butternut squash, peeled and diced
2 carrots, diced
1 cup dried green or brown lentils, rinsed
6 cups vegetable broth
1 can (15 oz) diced tomatoes
1 teaspoon ground cumin
1 teaspoon ground coriander
1/2 teaspoon ground turmeric
1/2 teaspoon paprika
Salt and pepper to taste
2 cups fresh spinach, chopped

Directions:
In a large pot, heat the olive oil over medium heat. Add the chopped onion and garlic, and sauté until the onion is translucent, about 5 minutes. Add the diced butternut squash and carrots, and cook for another 5 minutes, stirring occasionally.
Stir in the lentils, vegetable broth, diced tomatoes, ground cumin, ground coriander, ground turmeric, paprika, salt, and pepper. Bring the mixture to a boil, then reduce the heat and let it simmer for about 30 minutes, or until the lentils and vegetables are tender. Stir in the chopped spinach and cook for an additional 5 minutes until wilted.
Serve hot, garnished with fresh cilantro if desired.

Fresh Spring Rolls with Peanut Dipping Sauce

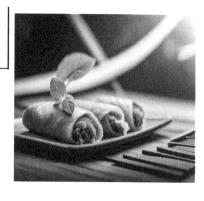

Prepping Time: 25 minutes
Cooking Time: 0 minutes
Portion Size: 4 servings

Nutritional Data: 280 calories
Protein: 8g | Fat: 12g
Carbohydrates: 36g | Fiber: 4g
Sugar: 8g | Sodium: 700 mg

Ingredients:
For the Spring Rolls:
8 rice paper wrappers
1 cup shredded carrots
1 cup thinly sliced red bell pepper
1 cup thinly sliced cucumber
1 cup shredded purple cabbage
1 cup cooked vermicelli rice noodles
1 cup fresh mint leaves
1 cup fresh cilantro leaves
1 cup fresh basil leaves
For the Peanut Dipping Sauce:
1/4 cup creamy peanut butter
2 tablespoons soy sauce or tamari
1 tablespoon hoisin sauce
1 tablespoon fresh lime juice
1 garlic clove, minced
1 teaspoon grated fresh ginger
2-3 tablespoons warm water (to thin the sauce)

Directions:
Prepare all the vegetables and herbs, setting them aside in separate bowls. Fill a large bowl with warm water. Dip one rice paper wrapper into the warm water for about 10-15 seconds, until soft and pliable. Remove from the water and lay flat on a clean surface. In the center of the wrapper, place a small handful of carrots, red bell pepper, cucumber, purple cabbage, vermicelli rice noodles, mint leaves, cilantro leaves, and basil leaves. Fold the bottom of the wrapper over the filling, then fold in the sides, and roll tightly. Repeat with the remaining wrappers and fillings. For the peanut dipping sauce, combine the peanut butter, soy sauce or tamari, hoisin sauce, lime juice, minced garlic, and grated ginger in a bowl. Mix well. Add warm water a tablespoon at a time until the sauce reaches your desired consistency. Serve the spring rolls with the peanut dipping sauce on the side.

Veggie-Packed Quinoa Patties with Avocado Sauce

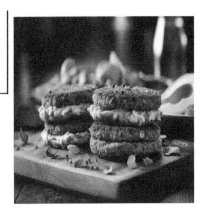

Prepping Time: 20 minutes
Cooking Time: 20 minutes
Portion Size: 4 servings

Nutritional Data: 320 calories
Protein: 12g | Fat: 18g
Carbohydrates: 28g | Fiber: 8g
Sugar: 4g | Sodium: 280 mg

Ingredients:
For the Quinoa Patties:
1 cup cooked quinoa
1 cup grated zucchini
1 cup grated carrot
1/2 cup chopped spinach
1/4 cup chopped red onion
2 cloves garlic, minced
2 eggs, beaten
1/4 cup breadcrumbs
1/4 cup grated Parmesan cheese (optional)
1 teaspoon dried oregano
Salt and pepper to taste
2 tablespoons olive oil
For the Avocado Sauce:
1 ripe avocado
1/4 cup Greek yogurt
1 tablespoon lime juice
1 clove garlic, minced
Salt and pepper to taste

Directions:
In a large bowl, combine the cooked quinoa, grated zucchini, grated carrot, chopped spinach, chopped red onion, minced garlic, beaten eggs, breadcrumbs, Parmesan cheese (if using), dried oregano, salt, and pepper. Mix until well combined.
Form the mixture into patties. In a large skillet, heat the olive oil over medium heat. Cook the patties for about 4-5 minutes on each side, or until golden brown and cooked through. While the patties are cooking, prepare the avocado sauce. In a blender or food processor, combine the avocado, Greek yogurt, lime juice, minced garlic, salt, and pepper. Blend until smooth.
Serve the quinoa patties hot with a dollop of avocado sauce on top.

Turmeric-Spiced Lentil and Rice Pilaf

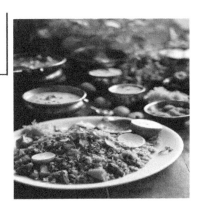

Prepping Time: 10 minutes
Cooking Time: 30 minutes
Portion Size: 4 servings

Nutritional Data: 320 calories
Protein: 10g | Fat: 8g
Carbohydrates: 50g | Fiber: 10g
Sugar: 3g | Sodium: 400 mg

Ingredients:
1 tablespoon olive oil
1 medium onion, finely chopped
2 garlic cloves, minced
1 cup basmati rice
1 cup dried green or brown lentils, rinsed
1 teaspoon ground turmeric
1 teaspoon ground cumin
1/2 teaspoon ground coriander
1/2 teaspoon ground cinnamon
4 cups vegetable broth
1/2 cup chopped fresh parsley
1/4 cup slivered almonds (optional)
Salt and pepper to taste
Lemon wedges for serving

Directions:
In a large pot, heat the olive oil over medium heat. Add the chopped onion and garlic, and sauté until the onion is translucent, about 5 minutes. Stir in the rice, lentils, turmeric, cumin, coriander, and cinnamon. Cook for 2-3 minutes, stirring frequently, until the spices are fragrant. Pour in the vegetable broth, bring to a boil, then reduce the heat to low, cover, and simmer for about 25-30 minutes, or until the rice and lentils are tender and the liquid is absorbed.
Fluff the pilaf with a fork and stir in the chopped parsley and slivered almonds if using. Season with salt and pepper to taste.
Serve hot, garnished with lemon wedges.

Roasted Beet and Arugula Salad with Walnuts

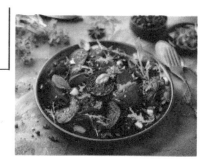

Prepping Time: 15 minutes
Cooking Time: 40 minutes
Portion Size: 4 servings

Nutritional Data: 250 calories
Protein: 6g | Fat: 16g
Carbohydrates: 22g | Fiber: 5g
Sugar: 13g | Sodium: 150 mg

Ingredients:
4 medium beets, scrubbed and trimmed
1 tablespoon olive oil
Salt and pepper to taste
4 cups fresh arugula
1/2 cup crumbled goat cheese (optional)
1/4 cup walnuts, toasted
1/4 cup balsamic vinegar
1 tablespoon honey or maple syrup
1/4 cup extra-virgin olive oil

Directions:
Preheat the oven to 400°F (200°C). Wrap each beet individually in aluminum foil and place them on a baking sheet. Roast for about 40 minutes, or until the beets are tender when pierced with a fork. Allow the beets to cool slightly, then peel and cut them into wedges. In a small bowl, whisk together the balsamic vinegar, honey or maple syrup, and extra-virgin olive oil. Season with salt and pepper to taste. In a large bowl, combine the arugula, roasted beet wedges, crumbled goat cheese (if using), and toasted walnuts. Drizzle the salad with the balsamic dressing and toss gently to combine.
Serve immediately and enjoy your nutritious roasted beet and arugula salad.

Broccoli and Almond Stir-Fry with Brown Rice

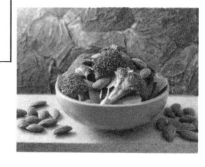

Prepping Time: 10 minutes
Cooking Time: 20 minutes
Portion Size: 4 servings

Nutritional Data: 350 calories
Protein: 10g | Fat: 14g
Carbohydrates: 48g | Fiber: 7g
Sugar: 5g | Sodium: 480 mg

Ingredients:
1 cup brown rice
2 cups water
2 tablespoons olive oil
1 large head of broccoli, cut into florets
1 red bell pepper, thinly sliced
2 garlic cloves, minced
1-inch piece of ginger, minced
1/4 cup low-sodium soy sauce or tamari
2 tablespoons hoisin sauce (optional)
1/4 cup sliced almonds, toasted
2 green onions, chopped
1 tablespoon sesame seeds (optional)
Salt and pepper to taste

Directions:
In a medium saucepan, bring the brown rice and water to a boil. Reduce heat to low, cover, and simmer for about 40-45 minutes, or until the rice is tender and the water is absorbed. Fluff with a fork and set aside.
While the rice is cooking, heat the olive oil in a large skillet or wok over medium-high heat. Add the minced garlic and ginger, and sauté for about 1 minute until fragrant.
Add the broccoli florets and red bell pepper to the skillet. Stir-fry for about 5-7 minutes, or until the vegetables are tender-crisp. Stir in the soy sauce or tamari and hoisin sauce (if using). Cook for another 2-3 minutes, stirring frequently, until the vegetables are well-coated with the sauce.
Add the toasted almonds and chopped green onions to the skillet. Toss to combine and season with salt and pepper to taste.
Serve the stir-fry over the cooked brown rice, garnished with sesame seeds if desired.

DINNER RECIPES

Roasted Vegetable and Quinoa Stuffed Peppers

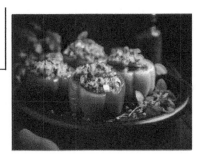

Prepping Time: 15 minutes
Cooking Time: 40 minutes
Portion Size: 4 servings

Nutritional Data: 290 calories
Protein: 10g | Fat: 10g
Carbohydrates: 40g | Fiber: 7g
Sugar: 8g | Sodium: 350 mg

Ingredients:
4 large bell peppers, tops cut off and seeds removed
1 cup quinoa, rinsed
2 cups vegetable broth
1 zucchini, diced
1 yellow squash, diced
1 red bell pepper, diced
1/2 red onion, diced
1 tablespoon olive oil
1 teaspoon dried oregano
1 teaspoon dried basil
Salt and pepper to taste

Directions:
Preheat the oven to 400°F (200°C). Place the bell peppers cut side up in a baking dish.
In a medium saucepan, bring the vegetable broth to a boil. Add the quinoa, reduce heat, cover, and simmer for about 15 minutes, or until the quinoa is tender and the liquid is absorbed. Fluff with a fork and set aside. While the quinoa is cooking, toss the diced zucchini, yellow squash, red bell pepper, and red onion with olive oil, oregano, basil, salt, and pepper. Spread the vegetables on a baking sheet and roast in the preheated oven for 20 minutes, or until tender. In a large bowl, combine the cooked quinoa and roasted vegetables. Stir in the crumbled feta cheese if using. Spoon the quinoa and vegetable mixture into the prepared bell peppers, packing it in tightly. Cover the baking dish with foil and bake for 20 minutes. Remove the foil and bake for an additional 10 minutes, or until the peppers are tender. Garnish with fresh parsley if desired. Serve immediately and enjoy

Lentil and Sweet Potato Shepherd's Pie

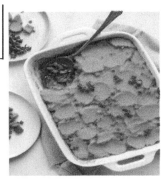

Prepping Time: 20 minutes
Cooking Time: 40 minutes
Portion Size: 6 servings

Nutritional Data: 350 calories
Protein: 12g | Fat: 8g
Carbohydrates: 58g | Fiber: 14g
Sugar: 12g | Sodium: 400 mg

Ingredients:
For the Filling:
1 tablespoon olive oil
1 large onion, chopped
2 garlic cloves, minced
2 large carrots, diced
2 celery stalks, diced
1 cup dried green or brown lentils, rinsed
4 cups vegetable broth
1 can (15 oz) diced tomatoes
1 teaspoon dried thyme
1 teaspoon dried rosemary
Salt and pepper to taste
1 cup frozen peas
For the Sweet Potato Topping:
4 large sweet potatoes, peeled and cubed
1/4 cup unsweetened almond milk
2 tablespoons olive oil - Salt and pepper to taste

Directions:
Preheat the oven to 375°F (190°C). In a large pot, heat the olive oil over medium heat. Add the onion and garlic, and sauté until the onion is translucent, about 5 minutes. Add the carrots and celery, and cook for another 5 minutes until they begin to soften. Stir in the lentils, vegetable broth, diced tomatoes, thyme, rosemary, salt, and pepper. Bring to a boil, then reduce the heat and simmer for about 25 minutes, or until the lentils are tender and the mixture has thickened. Stir in the frozen peas and cook for an additional 5 minutes. While the lentil mixture is simmering, place the sweet potatoes in a large pot and cover with water. Bring to a boil and cook until the sweet potatoes are tender, about 15 minutes. Drain and return to the pot. Add the almond milk, olive oil, salt, and pepper to the sweet potatoes. Mash until smooth and creamy. Spread the lentil mixture evenly in a large baking dish. Spoon the mashed sweet potatoes over the top and spread evenly. Bake in the preheated oven until the top is golden. Serve Hot

Cauliflower Steak with Chimichurri Sauce

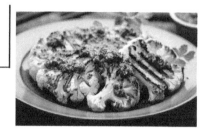

Prepping Time: 15 minutes
Cooking Time: 25 minutes
Portion Size: 4 servings

Nutritional Data: 220 calories
Protein: 3g | Fat: 20g
Carbohydrates: 10g | Fiber: 4g
Sugar: 2g | Sodium: 300 mg

Ingredients:
For the Cauliflower Steaks:
1 large head of cauliflower
2 tablespoons olive oil
1 teaspoon smoked paprika
1/2 teaspoon garlic powder
Salt and pepper to taste
For the Chimichurri Sauce:
1 cup fresh parsley, finely chopped
1/2 cup fresh cilantro, finely chopped
1/4 cup red wine vinegar
1/2 cup olive oil
3 garlic cloves, minced
1 teaspoon red pepper flakes (optional)
Salt and pepper to taste

Directions:
Preheat the oven to 400°F (200°C). Line a baking sheet with parchment paper.
Remove the leaves and trim the stem of the cauliflower, keeping the core intact. Slice the cauliflower into 1-inch thick steaks. You should get about 4 steaks from one large head of cauliflower. In a small bowl, mix the olive oil, smoked paprika, garlic powder, salt, and pepper. Brush both sides of the cauliflower steaks with the seasoned olive oil.
Place the cauliflower steaks on the prepared baking sheet and roast for 20-25 minutes, flipping halfway through, until tender and golden brown. While the cauliflower is roasting, prepare the chimichurri sauce. In a medium bowl, combine the chopped parsley, cilantro, red wine vinegar, olive oil, minced garlic, red pepper flakes (if using), salt, and pepper. Stir well to combine.
Once the cauliflower steaks are done, remove them from the oven and transfer to serving plates.
Spoon the chimichurri sauce over the cauliflower steaks and serve immediately.

Spicy Chickpea and Spinach Curry

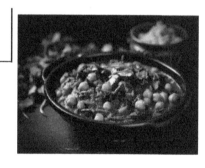

Prepping Time: 10 minutes
Cooking Time: 30 minutes
Portion Size: 4 servings

Nutritional Data: 300 calories
Protein: 8g | Fat: 14g
Carbohydrates: 36g | Fiber: 8g
Sugar: 6g | Sodium: 480 mg

Ingredients:
1 tablespoon olive oil
1 large onion, finely chopped
3 garlic cloves, minced
1 tablespoon fresh ginger, grated
1 tablespoon curry powder
1 teaspoon ground cumin
1 teaspoon ground coriander
1/2 teaspoon ground turmeric
1/2 teaspoon cayenne pepper (adjust to taste)
1 can (15 oz) diced tomatoes
1 can (15 oz) coconut milk
1 can (15 oz) chickpeas, drained and rinsed
4 cups fresh spinach, chopped
Salt and pepper to taste
Fresh cilantro for garnish (optional)

Directions:
In a large pot, heat the olive oil over medium heat. Add the chopped onion and sauté until translucent, about 5 minutes.
Add the minced garlic and grated ginger, and sauté for another 2 minutes until fragrant.
Stir in the curry powder, ground cumin, ground coriander, ground turmeric, and cayenne pepper. Cook for 1-2 minutes, stirring constantly to toast the spices. Add the diced tomatoes and coconut milk to the pot, stirring well to combine. Bring the mixture to a simmer, then add the chickpeas. Simmer for about 15 minutes, allowing the flavors to meld and the curry to thicken slightly.
Stir in the chopped spinach and cook for an additional 5 minutes until wilted. Season with salt and pepper to taste.
Serve hot, garnished with fresh cilantro if desired.

Baked Salmon with Lemon-Dill Quinoa

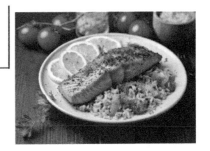

Prepping Time: 10 minutes
Cooking Time: 20 minutes
Portion Size: 4 servings

Nutritional Data: 420 calories
Protein: 30g | Fat: 20g
Carbohydrates: 30g | Fiber: 5g
Sugar: 2g | Sodium: 350 mg

Ingredients:
For the Salmon:
4 salmon fillets
2 tablespoons olive oil
1 lemon, thinly sliced
Salt and pepper to taste
For the Lemon-Dill Quinoa:
1 cup quinoa, rinsed
2 cups vegetable broth
1 tablespoon olive oil
2 tablespoons fresh dill, chopped
1 lemon, zested and juiced
Salt and pepper to taste

Directions:
Preheat the Oven: Preheat the oven to 375°F (190°C). Place the salmon fillets on a baking sheet lined with parchment paper.
Drizzle olive oil over the salmon and season with salt and pepper. Top each fillet with lemon slices.
Bake for 15-20 minutes, or until the salmon is cooked through and flakes easily with a fork.
In a medium saucepan, bring the vegetable broth to a boil. Add the quinoa, reduce heat, cover, and simmer for about 15 minutes, or until the quinoa is tender and the liquid is absorbed. Fluff with a fork. Stir in the olive oil, chopped dill, lemon zest, and lemon juice into the cooked quinoa. Season with salt and pepper to taste. Serve: Divide the lemon-dill quinoa among four plates. Top each serving with a baked salmon fillet. Garnish with additional fresh dill and lemon slices if desired.

Zucchini Lasagna with Cashew Ricotta

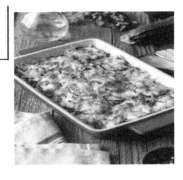

Prepping Time: 25 minutes
Cooking Time: 40 minutes
Portion Size: 6 servings

Nutritional Data: 320 calories
Protein: 10g | Fat: 18g
Carbohydrates: 32g | Fiber: 6g
Sugar: 10g | Sodium: 500 mg

Ingredients:
For the Lasagna:
4 medium zucchinis, thinly sliced lengthwise
2 cups marinara sauce
1 cup spinach leaves, chopped
1 cup mushrooms, sliced
1/2 cup onion, finely chopped
2 cloves garlic, minced
1 tablespoon olive oil
Salt and pepper to taste
For the Cashew Ricotta:
1 1/2 cups raw cashews, soaked in water for at least 2 hours
1/4 cup nutritional yeast
2 tablespoons lemon juice
1 garlic clove, minced
1/4 cup water
Salt and pepper to taste

Directions:
Prepare the Cashew Ricotta: Drain and rinse the soaked cashews. In a food processor, combine the cashews, nutritional yeast, lemon juice, minced garlic, and water. Blend until smooth and creamy. Season with salt and pepper to taste.
Prepare the Vegetables: In a large skillet, heat olive oil over medium heat. Add the chopped onion and minced garlic, and sauté until translucent, about 5 minutes. Add the sliced mushrooms and chopped spinach, cooking until tender. Season with salt and pepper. In a baking dish, spread a thin layer of marinara sauce. Place a layer of zucchini slices over the sauce.
Spread a layer of cashew ricotta over the zucchini slices. Add a layer of the sautéed vegetables. Repeat the layers until all ingredients are used, finishing with a layer of marinara sauce on top. Cover the dish with aluminum foil and bake for 30 minutes. Remove the foil and bake for an additional 10 minutes, or until the zucchini is tender and the top is slightly browned. Let the lasagna cool for a few minutes before slicing. Serve warm and enjoy

Eggplant and Mushroom Stir-Fry with Brown Rice

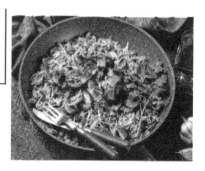

Prepping Time: 15 minutes
Cooking Time: 30 minutes
Portion Size: 4 servings

Nutritional Data: 280 calories
Protein: 6g | Fat: 12g
Carbohydrates: 38g | Fiber: 7g
Sugar: 8g | Sodium: 550 mg

Ingredients:
For the Stir-Fry:
1 cup brown rice and 2 cups water
2 tablespoons olive oil
1 large eggplant, diced
1 cup mushrooms, sliced
1 red bell pepper, sliced
1 onion, thinly sliced
2 cloves garlic, minced
1 tablespoon fresh ginger, minced
1/4 cup low-sodium soy sauce or tamari
2 tablespoons rice vinegar
1 tablespoon hoisin sauce (optional)
1 teaspoon sesame oil
1/4 cup fresh cilantro, chopped
2 green onions, chopped

Directions:
In a medium saucepan, bring the brown rice and water to a boil.
Reduce heat to low, cover, and simmer for about 40-45 minutes, or until the rice is tender and the water is absorbed. Fluff with a fork and set aside.
Prepare the Stir-Fry: In a large skillet or wok, heat olive oil over medium-high heat. Add the diced eggplant and cook for about 5-7 minutes until it begins to soften. Add the sliced mushrooms, red bell pepper, and onion. Stir-fry for another 5 minutes until the vegetables are tender. Stir in the minced garlic and fresh ginger, cooking for an additional 1-2 minutes until fragrant.
Add the soy sauce or tamari, rice vinegar, hoisin sauce (if using), and sesame oil. Stir well to combine and cook for another 2-3 minutes.
Serve: Divide the cooked brown rice among four plates. Top with the eggplant and mushroom stir-fry. Garnish with chopped fresh cilantro, green onions, and sesame seeds if desired. Serve immediately

Butternut Squash and Black Bean Enchiladas

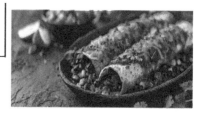

Prepping Time: 20 minutes
Cooking Time: 40 minutes
Portion Size: 4 servings

Nutritional Data: 350 calories
Protein: 12g | Fat: 10g
Carbohydrates: 58g | Fiber: 12g
Sugar: 8g | Sodium: 500 mg

Ingredients:
1 medium butternut squash, peeled and diced
1 tablespoon olive oil
1 teaspoon ground cumin
1/2 teaspoon chili powder
Salt and pepper to taste
1 can (15 oz) black beans, drained and rinsed
8 small whole wheat tortillas
2 cups enchilada sauce
1 cup shredded dairy-free cheese (optional)
1/4 cup chopped fresh cilantro

Directions:
Preheat oven and prepare baking sheet: Preheat the oven to 400°F (200°C). Line a baking sheet with parchment paper.
Roast butternut squash: In a large bowl, toss the diced butternut squash with olive oil, ground cumin, chili powder, salt, and pepper. Spread the seasoned squash on the prepared baking sheet and roast for about 25-30 minutes, or until tender and slightly caramelized. Prepare filling: In a medium bowl, combine the roasted butternut squash and black beans. Assemble enchiladas: Spread 1/2 cup of the enchilada sauce over the bottom of a 9x13-inch baking dish. Fill each tortilla with the butternut squash and black bean mixture, then roll up and place seam-side down in the baking dish. Repeat with remaining tortillas and filling.
Add sauce and cheese: Pour the remaining enchilada sauce over the top of the rolled tortillas. Sprinkle with shredded dairy-free cheese if using. Bake enchiladas: Cover the baking dish with foil and bake in the preheated oven for 15 minutes. Remove the foil and bake for an additional 10 minutes, or until the cheese is melted and bubbly. Garnish and serve: Remove from the oven and let cool for a few minutes. Garnish with chopped fresh cilantro and avocado slices if desired. Serve immediately.

Herb-Crusted Tofu with Roasted Brussels Sprouts

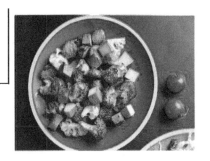

Prepping Time: 15 minutes
Cooking Time: 30 minutes
Portion Size: 4 servings

Nutritional Data: 320 calories
Protein: 14g | Fat: 18g
Carbohydrates: 26g | Fiber: 8g
Sugar: 5g | Sodium: 350 mg

Ingredients:
1 block (14 oz) firm tofu, drained and pressed
2 tablespoons olive oil
1 tablespoon fresh thyme, chopped
1 tablespoon fresh rosemary, chopped
1 tablespoon fresh parsley, chopped
2 garlic cloves, minced
Salt and pepper to taste
1 lb Brussels sprouts, trimmed and halved
1 tablespoon balsamic vinegar

Directions:
Preheat oven and prepare tofu: Preheat the oven to 400°F (200°C). Cut the pressed tofu into 1-inch cubes.
Season tofu: In a small bowl, mix together 1 tablespoon of olive oil, fresh thyme, rosemary, parsley, minced garlic, salt, and pepper. Toss the tofu cubes in the herb mixture until well-coated.
Prepare Brussels sprouts: In a separate bowl, toss the halved Brussels sprouts with the remaining 1 tablespoon of olive oil, balsamic vinegar, salt, and pepper.
Arrange on baking sheet: Spread the tofu cubes and Brussels sprouts on a large baking sheet lined with parchment paper, keeping them separate. Roast: Roast in the preheated oven for 25-30 minutes, stirring halfway through, until the tofu is golden and the Brussels sprouts are tender and caramelized. Remove from the oven and serve immediately.

Mediterranean Chickpea and Spinach Sauté

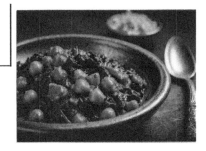

Prepping Time: 20 minutes
Cooking Time: 15 minutes
Portion Size: 4 servings

Nutritional Data: 220 calories
Protein: 8g | Fat: 10g
Carbohydrates: 24g | Fiber: 6g
Sugar: 5g | Sodium: 400 mg

Ingredients:
2 tablespoons olive oil
1 medium onion, chopped
3 garlic cloves, minced
1 can (15 oz) chickpeas, drained and rinsed
1 can (14.5 oz) diced tomatoes, drained
6 cups fresh spinach leaves
1 teaspoon dried oregano
1/2 teaspoon dried thyme
Salt and pepper to taste
1/4 cup crumbled feta cheese (optional)
Fresh parsley, chopped (for garnish)
Lemon wedges (for serving)

Directions:
In a large skillet, heat the olive oil over medium heat.
Add the chopped onion and sauté for about 5 minutes, until translucent.
Stir in the minced garlic and cook for another minute, until fragrant.
Add the chickpeas and diced tomatoes to the skillet, stirring to combine.
Season with dried oregano, dried thyme, salt, and pepper. Cook for about 5 minutes, allowing the flavors to meld.
Add the fresh spinach leaves, stirring until wilted, about 2-3 minutes.
Remove from heat and sprinkle with crumbled feta cheese, if using.
Garnish with fresh parsley and serve with lemon wedges.
Serve immediately and enjoy your nutritious Mediterranean Chickpea and Spinach Sauté.

Quinoa and Vegetable Stuffed Cabbage Rolls

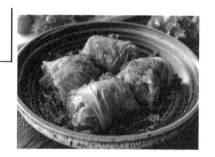

Prepping Time: 20 minutes
Cooking Time: 45 minutes
Portion Size: 4 servings

Nutritional Data: 280 calories
Protein: 8g | Fat: 8g
Carbohydrates: 46g | Fiber: 10g
Sugar: 10g | Sodium: 520 mg

Ingredients:
1 large head of cabbage
1 cup quinoa, rinsed
2 cups vegetable broth
1 tablespoon olive oil
1 small onion, chopped
2 garlic cloves, minced
1 carrot, grated
1 zucchini, grated
1 red bell pepper, diced
1 cup chopped spinach
1 teaspoon dried oregano
1 teaspoon dried basil
Salt and pepper to taste
2 cups marinara sauce
Fresh parsley, chopped (for garnish)

Directions:
In a large pot, bring water to a boil. Carefully add the cabbage and cook for about 5 minutes until the outer leaves are tender. Remove the cabbage and allow it to cool slightly. Gently separate 8 large leaves and set aside. In a medium saucepan, bring the vegetable broth to a boil. Add the quinoa, reduce heat, cover, and simmer for about 15 minutes, or until the quinoa is tender and the liquid is absorbed. Fluff with a fork and set aside. In a large skillet, heat the olive oil over medium heat. Add the onion and garlic, and sauté for about 5 minutes until translucent. Stir in the grated carrot, grated zucchini, red bell pepper, and chopped spinach. Cook for another 5 minutes until the vegetables are tender. Add the cooked quinoa to the skillet, along with the dried oregano, dried basil, salt, and pepper. Stir to combine and cook for another 2 minutes. Remove from heat. Preheat the oven to 375°F (190°C). Spread 1 cup of marinara sauce in the bottom of a large baking dish. Place about 1/4 cup of the quinoa mixture in the center of each cabbage leaf. Roll up the leaf, tucking in the sides to secure the filling. Place the rolls seam-side down in the baking dish. Pour the remaining marinara sauce over the cabbage rolls. Cover the dish with foil.
Bake for 30 minutes, or until the cabbage is tender and the filling is heated through. Garnish with fresh parsley and serve

Spaghetti with Zucchini Noodles and Pesto

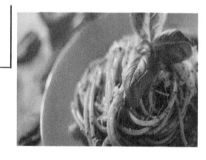

Prepping Time: 15 minutes
Cooking Time: 10 minutes
Portion Size: 4 servings

Nutritional Data: 400 calories
Protein: 12g | Fat: 20g
Carbohydrates: 46g | Fiber: 8g
Sugar: 5g | Sodium: 220 mg

Ingredients:
8 oz whole wheat spaghetti
2 large zucchinis, spiralized into noodles
1 cup fresh basil leaves
1/4 cup pine nuts
1/2 cup grated Parmesan cheese
2 garlic cloves
1/2 cup olive oil
Salt and pepper to taste
Cherry tomatoes for garnish (optional)

Directions:
Cook the whole wheat spaghetti according to package instructions until al dente. Drain and set aside.
In a food processor, combine basil leaves, pine nuts, grated Parmesan cheese, and garlic cloves. Pulse until finely chopped.
With the food processor running, slowly add the olive oil until the mixture is smooth and creamy. Season with salt and pepper to taste.
In a large skillet, lightly sauté the zucchini noodles over medium heat for about 2-3 minutes until just tender.
Add the cooked spaghetti to the skillet and toss gently to combine.
Pour the pesto sauce over the spaghetti and zucchini noodles, tossing to coat evenly.
Serve immediately, garnished with cherry tomatoes if desired.

Turmeric and Ginger Lentil Soup

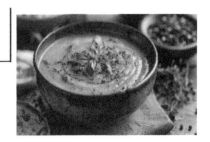

Prepping Time: 10 minutes
Cooking Time: 30 minutes
Portion Size: 4 servings

Nutritional Data: 220 calories
Protein: 10g | Fat: 5g
Carbohydrates: 35g | Fiber: 12g
Sugar: 6g | Sodium: 700 mg

Ingredients:
1 tablespoon olive oil
1 medium onion, chopped
2 garlic cloves, minced
1 tablespoon fresh ginger, grated
1 teaspoon ground turmeric
1 teaspoon ground cumin
1 cup red lentils, rinsed
4 cups vegetable broth
1 can (15 oz) diced tomatoes
1 carrot, diced
1 celery stalk, diced
1 teaspoon salt
1/2 teaspoon black pepper
1/4 teaspoon cayenne pepper (optional)
2 cups spinach leaves, chopped
Juice of 1 lemon and fresh cilantro for garnish

Directions:
In a large pot, heat the olive oil over medium heat. Add the chopped onion and cook until translucent, about 5 minutes.
Add the minced garlic and grated ginger, and sauté for another 2 minutes. Stir in the ground turmeric and ground cumin, and cook for 1 minute until fragrant. Add the rinsed red lentils, vegetable broth, diced tomatoes, carrot, celery, salt, black pepper, and cayenne pepper (if using). Bring to a boil. Reduce the heat to low and simmer for about 20 minutes, or until the lentils and vegetables are tender. Stir in the chopped spinach and cook for an additional 2-3 minutes until wilted.
Remove from heat and stir in the lemon juice. Serve hot, garnished with fresh cilantro.

Moroccan-Spiced Vegetable Tagine

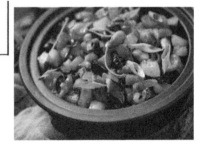

Prepping Time: 15 minutes
Cooking Time: 45 minutes
Portion Size: 4 servings

Nutritional Data: 320 calories
Protein: 8g | Fat: 8g
Carbohydrates: 58g | Fiber: 12g
Sugar: 16g | Sodium: 540 mg

Ingredients:
2 tablespoons olive oil
1 large onion, chopped
3 garlic cloves, minced
2 teaspoons ground cumin
2 teaspoons ground cinnamon
1 teaspoon ground turmeric
1 teaspoon ground ginger
2 large carrots, sliced
1 large sweet potato, peeled and cubed
1 zucchini, sliced
1 red bell pepper, chopped
1 can (15 oz) chickpeas, drained and rinsed
1 can (14.5 oz) diced tomatoes
1 cup vegetable broth
1/2 cup dried apricots, chopped
1/4 cup chopped fresh cilantro
Salt and pepper to taste
Cooked couscous or rice, for serving

Directions:
Heat the olive oil in a large pot or tagine over medium heat. Add the chopped onion and sauté until translucent, about 5 minutes.
Add the minced garlic, ground cumin, ground cinnamon, ground turmeric, ground ginger, and ground cayenne pepper (if using).
Stir well to combine and cook for another 1-2 minutes until fragrant. Add the sliced carrots, cubed sweet potato, sliced zucchini, and chopped red bell pepper to the pot. Stir to coat the vegetables with the spices. Add the drained chickpeas, diced tomatoes with their juice, vegetable broth, and chopped dried apricots. Stir well to combine. Bring the mixture to a boil, then reduce the heat to low and cover the pot. Simmer for 30-35 minutes, or until the vegetables are tender and the flavors have melded together.
Season with salt and pepper to taste. Stir in the chopped fresh cilantro just before serving. Serve the vegetable tagine over cooked couscous or rice.

Spinach and Mushroom Stuffed Portobello Mushrooms

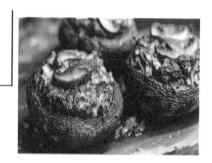

Prepping Time: 20 minutes
Cooking Time: 25 minutes
Portion Size: 4 servings

Nutritional Data: 180 calories
Protein: 7g | Fat: 10g
Carbohydrates: 15g | Fiber: 5g
Sugar: 3g | Sodium: 320 mg

Ingredients:
4 large portobello mushrooms, stems removed and gills scraped
2 tablespoons olive oil, divided
1 small onion, finely chopped
3 cloves garlic, minced
2 cups fresh spinach, chopped
1 cup button mushrooms, finely chopped
1/4 cup breadcrumbs (for a gluten-free option)
1/4 cup grated Parmesan cheese
Salt and pepper to taste
Fresh parsley, chopped for garnish

Directions:
Preheat the oven to 375°F (190°C). Line a baking sheet with parchment paper. Brush the portobello mushrooms with 1 tablespoon of olive oil on both sides. Place them on the prepared baking sheet, gill side up, and bake for 10 minutes. While the mushrooms are baking, heat the remaining 1 tablespoon of olive oil in a large skillet over medium heat. Add the onion and garlic, sautéing until fragrant and softened, about 5 minutes. Add the chopped button mushrooms to the skillet and cook until they release their moisture and become tender, about 5-7 minutes. Stir in the chopped spinach and cook until wilted, about 2 minutes. Season with salt, pepper, and red pepper flakes (if using). Remove the skillet from heat and stir in the breadcrumbs and Parmesan cheese (or nutritional yeast). Mix well. Remove the portobello mushrooms from the oven and fill each one with the spinach and mushroom mixture. Return the stuffed mushrooms to the oven and bake for an additional 15 minutes, or until the filling is heated through and the tops are golden brown. Garnish with chopped fresh parsley before serving.

Mixed Bean Salad with Fresh Herbs

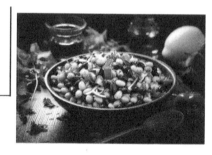

Prepping Time: 15 minutes
Cooking Time: 0 minutes
Portion Size: 4 servings

Nutritional Data: 210 calories
Protein: 8g | Fat: 7g
Carbohydrates: 30g | Fiber: 10g
Sugar: 4g | Sodium: 280 mg

Ingredients:

1 can (15 oz) black beans, drained and rinsed
1 can (15 oz) kidney beans, drained and rinsed
1 can (15 oz) chickpeas, drained and rinsed
1 small red onion, finely chopped
1 red bell pepper, diced
1 yellow bell pepper, diced
1 cucumber, diced
1/4 cup fresh parsley, chopped
1/4 cup fresh cilantro, chopped
1/4 cup fresh mint, chopped
3 tablespoons olive oil
2 tablespoons apple cider vinegar
Juice of 1 lemon
Salt and pepper to taste

Directions:
In a large bowl, combine the black beans, kidney beans, chickpeas, red onion, red bell pepper, yellow bell pepper, and cucumber. Add the chopped parsley, cilantro, and mint to the bowl. In a small bowl, whisk together the olive oil, apple cider vinegar, lemon juice, salt, and pepper. Pour the dressing over the bean mixture and toss to combine.
Serve immediately or refrigerate for an hour to let the flavors meld. Enjoy your refreshing Mixed Bean Salad with Fresh Herbs!

Cauliflower Rice Stir-Fry with Tofu

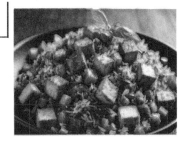

Prepping Time: 15 minutes
Cooking Time: 20 minutes
Portion Size: 4 servings

Nutritional Data: 220 calories
Protein: 12g | Fat: 14g
Carbohydrates: 12g | Fiber: 5g
Sugar: 3g | Sodium: 450 mg

Ingredients:

1 block (14 oz) firm tofu, drained and cubed
4 cups cauliflower rice
1 red bell pepper, diced
1 cup snap peas, trimmed and halved
1 carrot, julienned
1 small onion, finely chopped
2 cloves garlic, minced
1 tablespoon fresh ginger, minced
3 tablespoons soy sauce (or tamari for gluten-free)
1 tablespoon sesame oil
2 tablespoons olive oil
2 tablespoons sesame seeds
2 green onions, sliced
Salt and pepper to taste

Directions:

Place the tofu between paper towels and press it under a heavy object for about 10 minutes to remove excess water.
In a large skillet, heat 1 tablespoon of olive oil over medium-high heat. Add the cubed tofu and cook until golden brown on all sides, about 5-7 minutes. Remove from the skillet and set aside. In the same skillet, add the remaining olive oil. Sauté the onion, garlic, and ginger until fragrant, about 2 minutes. Add the red bell pepper, snap peas, and carrot to the skillet. Stir-fry for 5 minutes or until the vegetables are tender-crisp. Stir in the cauliflower rice and cook for another 5 minutes, until it is tender.
Combine tofu and sauce: Return the tofu to the skillet, pour in the soy sauce and sesame oil, and stir well to combine. Cook for an additional 2-3 minutes to heat everything through.Garnish and serve: Sprinkle with sesame seeds and sliced green onions. Adjust seasoning with salt and pepper to taste. Serve immediately and enjoy your healthy Cauliflower Rice Stir-Fry with Tofu!

Mediterranean Quinoa Salad & Lemon Vinaigrette

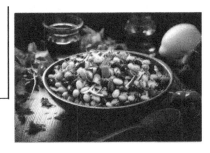

Prepping Time: 20 minutes
Cooking Time: 15 minutes
Portion Size: 4 servings

Nutritional Data: 290 calories
Protein: 8g | Fat: 14g
Carbohydrates: 34g | Fiber: 6g
Sugar: 3g | Sodium: 380 mg

Ingredients:
For the Salad:
1 cup quinoa, rinsed
2 cups water
1 cup cherry tomatoes, halved
1 cucumber, diced
1/2 red onion, finely chopped
1/2 cup Kalamata olives, pitted and sliced
1/4 cup fresh parsley, chopped
1/4 cup fresh mint, chopped
For the Lemon Vinaigrette:
1/4 cup extra-virgin olive oil
2 tablespoons freshly squeezed lemon juice
1 clove garlic, minced
1 teaspoon Dijon mustard
Salt and pepper to taste

Directions:
In a medium saucepan, bring the water to a boil. Add the quinoa, reduce the heat to low, cover, and simmer for about 15 minutes or until the quinoa has absorbed all the water. Remove from heat and let it sit, covered, for 5 minutes. Fluff with a fork and let it cool. While the quinoa is cooking, prepare the cherry tomatoes, cucumber, red onion, and Kalamata olives. Place them in a large salad bowl. Make the vinaigrette: In a small bowl, whisk together the extra-virgin olive oil, lemon juice, minced garlic, Dijon mustard, salt, and pepper until well combined. Add the cooled quinoa to the bowl with the vegetables. Pour the lemon vinaigrette over the salad and toss gently to combine. Add the crumbled feta cheese (if using), chopped parsley, and chopped mint. Toss again to mix everything well. Serve immediately or refrigerate for an hour to let the flavors meld together.

SNACKS AND SIDES

Spicy Roasted Chickpeas

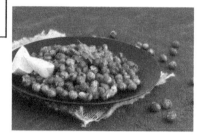

Prepping Time: 10 minutes
Cooking Time: 40 minutes
Portion Size: 4 servings

Nutritional Data: 120 calories
Protein: 6g | Fat: 5g
Carbohy8ates: 16g | Fiber: 5g
Sugar: 1g | Sodium: 230 mg

Ingredients:
1 can (15 oz) chickpeas, drained and rinsed
1 tablespoon olive oil
1 teaspoon smoked paprika
1/2 teaspoon ground cumin
1/2 teaspoon garlic powder
1/2 teaspoon onion powder
1/4 teaspoon cayenne pepper (adjust to taste)
Salt and pepper to taste

Directions:
Preheat the oven to 400°F (200°C). Line a baking sheet with parchment paper.
Pat the chickpeas dry with a paper towel, removing as much moisture as possible.
In a bowl, combine the chickpeas with olive oil, smoked paprika, ground cumin, garlic powder, onion powder, cayenne pepper, salt, and pepper. Toss until the chickpeas are evenly coated with the spices.
Spread the chickpeas in a single layer on the prepared baking sheet.
Roast in the preheated oven for 35-40 minutes, shaking the pan halfway through, until the chickpeas are crispy and golden brown.
Remove from the oven and let them cool slightly before serving.

Fresh Veggie Spring Rolls with Almond Sauce

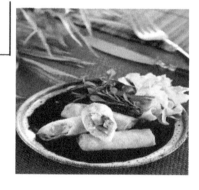

Prepping Time: 30 minutes
Cooking Time: 0 minutes
Portion Size: 4 servings

Nutritional Data: 180 calories
Protein: 6g | Fat: 9g
Carbohydrates: 20g | Fiber: 5g
Sugar: 5g | Sodium: 320 mg

Ingredients:
8 rice paper wrappers
1 cup thinly sliced carrots
1 cup thinly sliced cucumber
1 cup thinly sliced bell peppers
1 cup thinly sliced purple cabbage
1 cup fresh spinach leaves
1/4 cup fresh mint leaves
1/4 cup fresh cilantro leaves
For the Almond Sauce:
1/4 cup almond butter
2 tablespoons soy sauce (or tamari for gluten-free)
1 tablespoon lime juice
1 tablespoon maple syrup
1 teaspoon grated fresh ginger
1 garlic clove, minced
2-4 tablespoons warm water (to thin the sauce)
Instructions:

Directions:
Thinly slice all the vegetables and set them aside. Have the spinach, mint, and cilantro leaves ready.
In a bowl, whisk together almond butter, soy sauce, lime juice, maple syrup, grated ginger, and minced garlic. Add warm water, one tablespoon at a time, until the sauce reaches your desired consistency.
Fill a large shallow dish with warm water. Dip one rice paper wrapper into the water for about 10-15 seconds, until it becomes soft and pliable. Lay the softened wrapper on a clean surface.
Place a small amount of each vegetable, spinach, mint, and cilantro in the center of the wrapper. Fold the bottom of the wrapper over the filling, then fold in the sides, and roll tightly.
Serve the fresh veggie spring rolls immediately with the almond sauce on the side.

Quinoa and Black Bean Salad

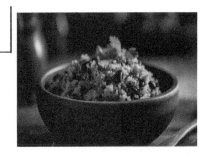

Prepping Time: 15 minutes
Cooking Time: 15 minutes
Portion Size: 4 servings

Nutritional Data: 320 calories
Protein: 10g | Fat: 14g
Carbohy8ates: 40g | Fiber: 10g
Sugar: 3g | Sodium: 400 mg

Ingredients:
1 cup quinoa
2 cups water
1 can (15 oz) black beans, rinsed and drained
1 cup cherry tomatoes, halved
1 red bell pepper, diced
1/2 cup red onion, finely chopped
1/2 cup fresh cilantro, chopped
1 avocado, diced
1/4 cup fresh lime juice
2 tablespoons olive oil
1 teaspoon ground cumin
Salt and pepper to taste

Directions:
In a medium saucepan, combine quinoa and water. Bring to a boil, then reduce heat to low, cover, and simmer for 15 minutes or until the quinoa is cooked and the water is absorbed. Fluff with a fork and let it cool. In a large bowl, combine the cooked quinoa, black beans, red bell pepper, yellow bell pepper, corn, red onion, and cilantro. In a small bowl, whisk together lime juice, olive oil, ground cumin, salt, and pepper. Pour the dressing over the quinoa mixture and toss to combine. Gently fold in the diced avocado. Serve immediately or refrigerate until ready to serve.

Turmeric-Spiced Roasted Cauliflower

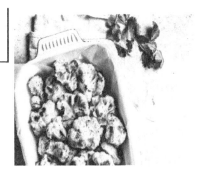

Prepping Time: 10 minutes
Cooking Time: 25 minutes
Portion Size: 4 servings

Nutritional Data: 120 calories
Protein: 3g | Fat: 7g
Carbohy8ates: 14g | Fiber: 5g
Sugar: 3g | Sodium: 200 mg

Ingredients:
1 large head of cauliflower, cut into florets
2 tablespoons olive oil
1 teaspoon ground turmeric
1/2 teaspoon ground cumin
1/2 teaspoon ground coriander
1/4 teaspoon cayenne pepper (optional, for heat)
Salt and pepper to taste
Fresh parsley, chopped (for garnish)
Lemon wedges (for serving)

Directions:
Preheat the oven to 425°F (220°C). Line a baking sheet with parchment paper.
In a large bowl, combine olive oil, turmeric, cumin, coriander, cayenne pepper, salt, and pepper.
Add the cauliflower florets to the bowl and toss until they are evenly coated with the spice mixture.
Spread the cauliflower florets in a single layer on the prepared baking sheet.
Roast in the preheated oven for 20-25 minutes, turning once halfway through, until the cauliflower is golden brown and tender.
Remove from the oven and transfer to a serving dish. Garnish with chopped fresh parsley and serve with lemon wedges.

Garlic and Herb Hummus with Carrot Sticks

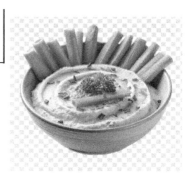

Prepping Time: 10 minutes
Cooking Time: 0 minutes
Portion Size: 4 servings

Nutritional Data: 180 calories
Protein: 6g | Fat: 10g
Carbohydrates: 18g | Fiber: 6g
Sugar: 4g | Sodium: 300 mg

Ingredients:
1 can (15 oz) chickpeas, drained and rinsed
2 tablespoons tahini
2 cloves garlic, minced
2 tablespoons fresh lemon juice
2 tablespoons olive oil
1 teaspoon ground cumin
1/2 teaspoon salt
1/4 teaspoon black pepper
2 tablespoons fresh parsley, chopped
2 tablespoons fresh cilantro, chopped
Water, as needed for desired consistency
4 large carrots, cut into sticks

Directions:
In a food processor, combine chickpeas, tahini, minced garlic, lemon juice, olive oil, ground cumin, salt, and black pepper.
Blend until smooth and creamy, adding water as needed to achieve the desired consistency.
Transfer the hummus to a serving bowl.
Stir in the chopped parsley and cilantro until well combined.
Serve the hummus with carrot sticks.

Zucchini Fritters with Yogurt Dip

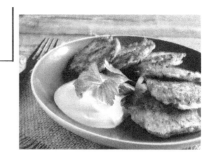

Prepping Time: 20 minutes
Cooking Time: 15 minutes
Portion Size: 4 servings

Nutritional Data: 150 calories
Protein: 7g | Fat: 8g
Carbohydrates: 12g | Fiber: 2g
Sugar: 3g | Sodium: 400 mg

Ingredients:
2 medium zucchinis, grated
1 teaspoon salt
1/4 cup all-purpose flour
1/4 cup grated Parmesan cheese
2 cloves garlic, minced
1 large egg, lightly beaten
1/2 teaspoon black pepper
2 tablespoons olive oil
Yogurt Dip:
1 cup Greek yogurt
1 tablespoon lemon juice
1 tablespoon fresh dill, chopped
Salt and pepper to taste

Directions:
Place grated zucchini in a colander and sprinkle with salt. Let it sit for 10 minutes, then squeeze out as much moisture as possible using a clean kitchen towel. In a large bowl, combine the zucchini, flour, Parmesan cheese, garlic, egg, and black pepper. Mix well to form a batter. Heat olive oil in a large skillet over medium heat. Scoop tablespoon-sized portions of the batter and drop them into the skillet, flattening them slightly with a spatula.
Cook the fritters for 3-4 minutes on each side, until golden brown and crispy. Transfer to a plate lined with paper towels to drain excess oil. In a small bowl, mix the Greek yogurt, lemon juice, fresh dill, salt, and pepper to make the yogurt dip.
Serve the zucchini fritters warm with the yogurt dip on the side.

Crispy Baked Tofu Bites

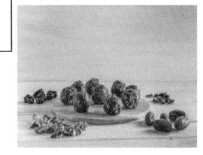

Prepping Time: 15 minutes
Cooking Time: 30 minutes
Portion Size: 4 servings

Nutritional Data: 140 calories
Protein: 10g | Fat: 8g
Carbohy8ates: 7g | Fiber: 1g
Sugar: 0g | Sodium: 320 mg

Ingredients:
1 block (14 oz) firm tofu, drained and pressed
2 tablespoons soy sauce
1 tablespoon olive oil
1 tablespoon cornstarch
1 teaspoon garlic powder
1 teaspoon smoked paprika
1/2 teaspoon black pepper

Directions:
Preheat the oven to 400°F (200°C). Line a baking sheet with parchment paper. Cut the pressed tofu into bite-sized cubes and place them in a large bowl. In a small bowl, mix the soy sauce and olive oil. Pour this mixture over the tofu cubes and gently toss to coat. In another bowl, combine the cornstarch, garlic powder, smoked paprika, and black pepper. Sprinkle this dry mixture over the tofu and toss again until evenly coated. Spread the tofu cubes in a single layer on the prepared baking sheet.
Bake in the preheated oven for 25-30 minutes, flipping halfway through, until the tofu is golden brown and crispy.
Remove from the oven and let cool slightly before serving. Enjoy as a snack or add to salads and stir-fries.

Raw Energy Balls with Dates and Nuts

Prepping Time: 15 minutes
Cooking Time: 0 minutes
Portion Size: 12 servings

Nutritional Data: 100 calories
Protein: 2g | Fat: 6g
Carbohydrates: 12g | Fiber: 2g
Sugar: 8g | Sodium: 10 mg

Ingredients:
1 cup pitted dates
1/2 cup almonds
1/2 cup walnuts
1/4 cup shredded coconut
2 tablespoons chia seeds
1 tablespoon cocoa powder
1 tablespoon coconut oil
1 teaspoon vanilla extract
A pinch of salt

Directions:
In a food processor, combine the pitted dates, almonds, walnuts, shredded coconut, chia seeds, cocoa powder, coconut oil, vanilla extract, and a pinch of salt.
Pulse the mixture until it forms a sticky dough-like consistency. If the mixture is too dry, add a small amount of water (1 teaspoon at a time) until the desired consistency is achieved.
Scoop out a tablespoon of the mixture and roll it into a ball. Repeat with the remaining mixture.
Place the energy balls on a plate and refrigerate for at least 30 minutes to firm up.
Store the energy balls in an airtight container in the refrigerator for up to two weeks.

Tomato and Basil Bruschetta on Whole Grain Bread

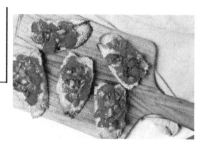

Prepping Time: 15 minutes
Cooking Time: 5 minutes
Portion Size: 4 servings

Nutritional Data: 180 calories
Protein: 5g | Fat: 8g
Carbohydrates: 22g | Fiber: 4g
Sugar: 5g | Sodium: 220 mg

Ingredients:
4 slices of whole grain bread
2 cups cherry tomatoes, diced
1/4 cup fresh basil leaves, chopped
2 cloves garlic, minced
2 tablespoons extra virgin olive oil
1 tablespoon balsamic vinegar
Salt and pepper to taste
1/4 cup grated Parmesan cheese (optional)

Directions:
Preheat the oven to 400°F (200°C). Arrange the bread slices on a baking sheet.
Toast the bread in the preheated oven for 5 minutes, or until golden and crispy.
In a bowl, combine the diced cherry tomatoes, chopped basil leaves, minced garlic, olive oil, balsamic vinegar, salt, and pepper. Mix well. Remove the toasted bread from the oven and let it cool slightly.
Spoon the tomato mixture evenly over the toasted bread slices. Optionally, sprinkle grated Parmesan cheese on top.
Serve immediately and enjoy your fresh Tomato and Basil Bruschetta.

Broccoli and Walnut Salad

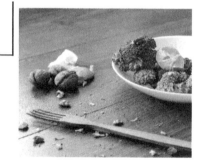

Prepping Time: 15 minutes
Cooking Time: 0 minutes
Portion Size: 4 servings

Nutritional Data: 180 calories
Protein: 6g | Fat: 10g
Carbohydrates: 18g | Fiber: 4g
Sugar: 9g | Sodium: 150 mg

Ingredients:
4 cups broccoli florets, finely chopped
1 cup shredded carrots
1/2 cup sliced walnuts, toasted
1/4 cup red onion, thinly sliced
1/4 cup dried cranberries
1/2 cup plain Greek yogurt
2 tablespoons apple cider vinegar
1 tablespoon honey
1 teaspoon Dijon mustard
Salt and pepper to taste

Directions:
In a large mixing bowl, combine the chopped broccoli florets, shredded carrots, toasted sliced walnuts, thinly sliced red onion, and dried cranberries. In a small bowl, whisk together the Greek yogurt, apple cider vinegar, honey, Dijon mustard, salt, and pepper until smooth and well combined.
Pour the dressing over the broccoli mixture and toss to coat evenly.
Serve immediately or refrigerate for up to 2 hours to allow the flavors to meld. Enjoy your nutritious Broccoli and Almond Slaw.

Avocado and Lime Guacamole with Veggie Chips

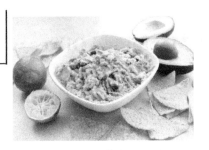

Prepping Time: 15 minutes
Cooking Time: 0 minutes
Portion Size: 4 servings

Nutritional Data: 200 calories
Protein: 2g | Fat: 18g
Carbohydrates: 12g | Fiber: 8g
Sugar: 2g | Sodium: 300 mg

Ingredients:
3 ripe avocados
1 lime, juiced
1/2 teaspoon salt
1/2 teaspoon ground cumin
1/2 teaspoon ground cayenne pepper
1/2 medium onion, finely diced
2 small tomatoes, diced
1 tablespoon chopped cilantro
1 clove garlic, minced
Veggie chips for serving

Directions:
Cut the avocados in half, remove the pit, and scoop the flesh into a mixing bowl.
Add the lime juice, salt, ground cumin, and cayenne pepper to the avocados.
Mash the mixture with a fork or potato masher until it reaches your desired consistency.
Fold in the diced onion, tomatoes, chopped cilantro, and minced garlic.
Serve immediately with veggie chips. Enjoy your fresh and nutritious Avocado and Lime Guacamole.

Cabbage and Carrot Sauerkraut

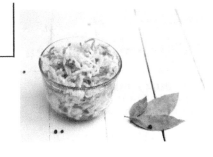

Prepping Time: 30 minutes
Cooking Time: 0 minutes
(fermentation time: 2-3 weeks)
Portion Size: 8 servings

Nutritional Data: 30 calories
Protein: 1g | Fat: 0g
Carbohydrates: 7g | Fiber: 3g
Sugar: 3g | Sodium: 400 mg

Ingredients:
1 medium head of green cabbage, shredded
2 large carrots, grated
1 tablespoon sea salt
1 tablespoon caraway seeds (optional)

Directions:
In a large mixing bowl, combine the shredded cabbage and grated carrots.
Sprinkle the sea salt over the vegetables and mix thoroughly. Let the mixture sit for about 10 minutes to allow the salt to draw out the moisture from the vegetables. Massage the mixture with your hands for about 5-10 minutes until it becomes soft and releases more liquid. If using, add the caraway seeds and mix well. Pack the mixture tightly into a clean, wide-mouth quart-sized mason jar, pressing down firmly to release any air pockets. Ensure the vegetables are submerged in their own liquid. If necessary, add a bit of water to cover them completely. Place a fermentation weight or a smaller jar filled with water on top of the vegetables to keep them submerged. Cover the jar with a clean cloth and secure it with a rubber band or string.
Store the jar in a cool, dark place for 2-3 weeks. Check daily to ensure the vegetables remain submerged and to remove any mold that may form on the surface. Taste the sauerkraut after 2 weeks. When it reaches your desired flavor, transfer it to the refrigerator to slow the fermentation process.

Marinated Olives with Lemon and Thyme

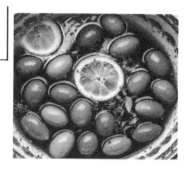

Prepping Time: 10 minutes
Cooking Time: 0 minutes
Portion Size: 8 servings

Nutritional Data: 110 calories
Protein: 1g | Fat: 11g
Carbohydrates: 2g | Fiber: 1g
Sugar: 0g | Sodium: 260 mg

Ingredients:
2 cups mixed olives (green and black)
1 lemon, zest and juice
3 sprigs fresh thyme
2 cloves garlic, thinly sliced
1/4 cup extra virgin olive oil
1/2 teaspoon red pepper flakes
Salt and black pepper to taste

Directions:
In a bowl, combine the mixed olives, lemon zest, lemon juice, fresh thyme sprigs, and sliced garlic.
Pour the extra virgin olive oil over the olive mixture.
Add the red pepper flakes, salt, and black pepper. Toss everything together until the olives are well coated.
Transfer the olives to a jar with a lid or an airtight container.
Marinate the olives in the refrigerator for at least 2 hours, preferably overnight, to allow the flavors to meld.
Before serving, bring the olives to room temperature. Enjoy as an appetizer or snack.

Edamame with Sea Salt and Lemon

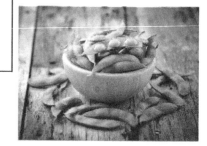

Prepping Time: 5 minutes
Cooking Time: 10 minutes
Portion Size: 4 servings

Nutritional Data: 120 calories
Protein: 1g | Fat: 5g
Carbohydrates: 9g | Fiber: 4g
Sugar: 2g | Sodium: 300 mg

Ingredients:
2 cups frozen edamame (in pods)
1 tablespoon sea salt
1 lemon, cut into wedges

Directions:
Bring a large pot of water to a boil.
Add the frozen edamame to the boiling water and cook for 5-7 minutes, or until the edamame are tender.
Drain the edamame and transfer them to a serving bowl.
Sprinkle the sea salt over the hot edamame and toss to coat evenly.
Serve with lemon wedges on the side. Squeeze lemon juice over the edamame just before eating for a burst of fresh flavor.

DESSERTS AND TREATS

Avocado Chocolate Mousse

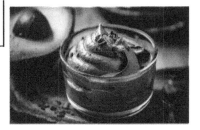

Prepping Time: 10 minutes
Cooking Time: 0 minutes
Portion Size: 4 servings

Nutritional Data: 210 calories
Protein: 3g | Fat: 14g
Carbohydrates: 23g | Fiber: 7g
Sugar: 13g | Sodium: 40 mg

Ingredients:
2 ripe avocados, peeled and pitted
1/4 cup unsweetened cocoa powder
1/4 cup maple syrup or honey
1/4 cup almond milk or any plant-based milk
1 teaspoon vanilla extract
A pinch of sea salt
Fresh berries and mint leaves for garnish (optional)

Directions:
In a food processor or blender, combine the avocados, cocoa powder, maple syrup, almond milk, vanilla extract, and sea salt.
Blend until smooth and creamy, scraping down the sides as needed to ensure all ingredients are well incorporated.
Taste and adjust the sweetness by adding more maple syrup or honey if desired.
Spoon the mousse into serving dishes and chill in the refrigerator for at least 30 minutes before serving.
Garnish with fresh berries and mint leaves if desired.
Serve chilled and enjoy!

Almond and Coconut Energy Bites

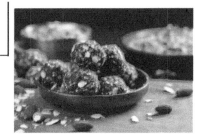

Prepping Time: 10 minutes
Cooking Time: 0 minutes
Portion Size: 12 bites

Nutritional Data: 150 calories
Protein: 4g | Fat: 9g
Carbohydrates: 15g | Fiber: 3g
Sugar: 10g | Sodium: 20 mg

Ingredients:
1 cup almonds
1 cup pitted dates
1/2 cup shredded unsweetened coconut
2 tablespoons chia seeds
2 tablespoons almond butter
1 tablespoon coconut oil
1 teaspoon vanilla extract
A pinch of sea salt

Directions:
In a food processor, combine the almonds, dates, shredded coconut, chia seeds, almond butter, coconut oil, vanilla extract, and sea salt. Pulse until the mixture is well combined and forms a sticky dough.
Using your hands, roll the mixture into small bite-sized balls.
Place the energy bites on a baking sheet lined with parchment paper and chill in the refrigerator for at least 30 minutes to set.
Store the energy bites in an airtight container in the refrigerator for up to one week.

Banana and Oatmeal Cookies

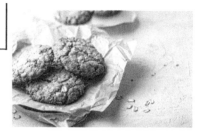

Prepping Time: 10 minutes
Cooking Time: 15 minutes
Portion Size: 12 cookies

Nutritional Data: 100 calories
Protein: 2g | Fat: 4g
Carbohydrates: 15g | Fiber: 2g
Sugar: 6g | Sodium: 30 mg

Ingredients:
2 ripe bananas, mashed
1 cup rolled oats
1/2 cup almond flour
1/4 cup almond butter
1/4 cup honey or maple syrup
1 teaspoon vanilla extract
1/2 teaspoon ground cinnamon
1/4 teaspoon baking powder
A pinch of salt
Optional: 1/4 cup dark chocolate chips or raisins

Directions:
Preheat the oven to 350°F (175°C). Line a baking sheet with parchment paper.
In a large bowl, combine the mashed bananas, rolled oats, almond flour, almond butter, honey (or maple syrup), vanilla extract, ground cinnamon, baking powder, and a pinch of salt. Mix until well combined.
Fold in the dark chocolate chips or raisins, if using.
Drop spoonfuls of the cookie dough onto the prepared baking sheet, flattening them slightly with the back of the spoon.
Bake in the preheated oven for 12-15 minutes, or until the cookies are golden brown and firm to the touch.
Allow the cookies to cool on the baking sheet for a few minutes before transferring them to a wire rack to cool completely!

Dark Chocolate and Walnut Brownies

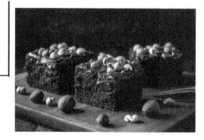

Prepping Time: 15 minutes
Cooking Time: 25 minutes
Portion Size: 12 servings

Nutritional Data: 210 calories
Protein: 4g | Fat: 15g
Carbohydrates: 18g | Fiber: 3g
Sugar: 12g | Sodium: 80 mg

Ingredients:
1 cup dark chocolate chips
1/2 cup coconut oil
1 cup coconut sugar
3 large eggs
1 teaspoon vanilla extract
1/2 cup almond flour
1/4 cup unsweetened cocoa powder
1/2 teaspoon baking powder
1/4 teaspoon salt
1/2 cup chopped walnuts

Directions:
Preheat the oven to 350°F (175°C). Line an 8x8 inch baking dish with parchment paper.
In a microwave-safe bowl, melt the dark chocolate chips and coconut oil together in 30-second intervals, stirring in between until smooth. Stir in the coconut sugar until well combined. Add the eggs one at a time, mixing well after each addition. Stir in the vanilla extract. In a separate bowl, whisk together the almond flour, cocoa powder, baking powder, and salt.
Gradually add the dry ingredients to the wet ingredients, stirring until just combined.
Fold in the chopped walnuts. Pour the batter into the prepared baking dish, spreading it out evenly.
Bake in the preheated oven for 20-25 minutes, or until a toothpick inserted into the center comes out with a few moist crumbs.
Allow the brownies to cool completely in the baking dish before lifting them out using the parchment paper and cutting them into squares.

Cashew and Date Bliss Balls

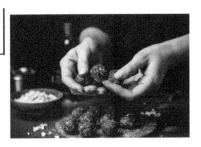

Prepping Time: 15 minutes
Cooking Time: 0 minutes
Portion Size: 12 servings

Nutritional Data: 150 calories
Protein: 3g | Fat: 9g
Carbohydrates: 18g | Fiber: 3g
Sugar: 14g | Sodium: 10 mg

Ingredients:
1 cup raw cashews
1 cup Medjool dates, pitted
1/2 cup unsweetened shredded coconut
1 tablespoon coconut oil
1 teaspoon vanilla extract
Pinch of salt

Directions:
In a food processor, combine the cashews and dates. Process until the mixture is finely chopped and begins to clump together.
Add the shredded coconut, coconut oil, vanilla extract, and a pinch of salt. Process again until well combined and the mixture starts to form a dough-like consistency.
Scoop out about a tablespoon of the mixture and roll it into a ball using your hands. Repeat with the remaining mixture.
Place the bliss balls on a plate or baking sheet and refrigerate for at least 30 minutes to firm up.
Store in an airtight container in the refrigerator for up to one week.

Berry and Almond Chia Pudding

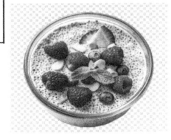

Prepping Time: 10 minutes
Cooking Time: 0 minutes
Portion Size: 4 servings

Nutritional Data: 180 calories
Protein: 5g | Fat: 9g
Carbohydrates: 21g | Fiber: 8g
Sugar: 9g | Sodium: 45 mg

Ingredients:
1 cup unsweetened almond milk
1/2 cup fresh or frozen mixed berries
1/4 cup chia seeds
2 tablespoons maple syrup or honey
1 teaspoon vanilla extract
1/4 cup sliced almonds
Fresh berries and mint leaves for garnish (optional)

Directions:
In a medium bowl, whisk together the almond milk, maple syrup (or honey), and vanilla extract.
Add the chia seeds and whisk until well combined.
Gently fold in the mixed berries. Cover the bowl and refrigerate for at least 4 hours or overnight, until the chia seeds have absorbed the liquid and the mixture has thickened. Before serving, stir the pudding to ensure even distribution of the chia seeds.
Spoon the chia pudding into serving bowls or jars. Top with sliced almonds, fresh berries, and mint leaves if desired.
Serve and enjoy!

Pumpkin Spice Energy Balls

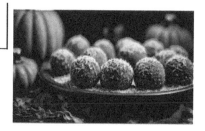

Prepping Time: 15 minutes
Cooking Time: 0 minutes
Portion Size: 12 servings

Nutritional Data: 110 calories
Protein: 3g | Fat: 5g
Carbohydrates: 14g | Fiber: 2g
Sugar: 6g | Sodium: 50 mg

Ingredients:
1 cup rolled oats
1/2 cup pumpkin puree
1/2 cup almond butter
1/4 cup honey or maple syrup
1/4 cup ground flaxseed
1/2 cup mini chocolate chips or raisins
1 teaspoon vanilla extract
1 teaspoon pumpkin pie spice
1/4 teaspoon salt

Directions:
In a large bowl, combine the rolled oats, pumpkin puree, almond butter, honey (or maple syrup), ground flaxseed, chocolate chips (or raisins), vanilla extract, pumpkin pie spice, and salt.
Stir until all the ingredients are well mixed and a sticky dough forms.
Using your hands, roll the mixture into 1-inch balls and place them on a baking sheet lined with parchment paper.
Refrigerate the energy balls for at least 30 minutes to allow them to firm up.
Once firm, transfer the energy balls to an airtight container. Store them in the refrigerator for up to a week.

Chocolate-Dipped Strawberries with Pistachios

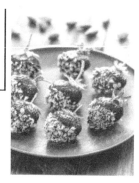

Prepping Time: 20 minutes
Cooking Time: 0 minutes
Portion Size: 12 servings

Nutritional Data: 70 calories
Protein: 1g | Fat: 4g
Carbohydrates: 8g | Fiber: 1g
Sugar: 6g | Sodium: 2 mg

Ingredients:
1 pound fresh strawberries, washed and dried
1 cup dark chocolate chips
1/2 cup shelled pistachios, finely chopped

Directions:
Line a baking sheet with parchment paper.
In a microwave-safe bowl, melt the dark chocolate chips in 30-second intervals, stirring between each interval until smooth.
Dip each strawberry into the melted chocolate, allowing the excess to drip off.
Roll the chocolate-coated strawberries in the chopped pistachios, ensuring an even coating.
Place the strawberries on the prepared baking sheet.
Refrigerate for at least 30 minutes or until the chocolate is set.
Serve chilled and enjoy!

Lemon and Blueberry Sorbet

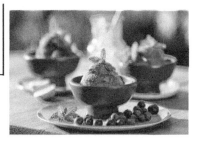

Prepping Time: 15 minutes
Cooking Time: 0 minutes
Portion Size: 4 servings

Nutritional Data: 80 calories
Protein: 0.5g | Fat: 0.1g
Carbohydrates: 21g | Fiber: 2g
Sugar: 17g | Sodium: 1 mg

Ingredients:
1 cup fresh blueberries
1/2 cup freshly squeezed lemon juice (about 2 lemons)
1/2 cup water
1/4 cup honey or maple syrup
1 teaspoon lemon zest

Directions:
In a blender, combine the blueberries, lemon juice, water, honey (or maple syrup), and lemon zest.
Blend until smooth.
Pour the mixture into a shallow, freezer-safe container.
Freeze for about 2-3 hours, stirring every 30 minutes to break up any ice crystals.
Once the sorbet is firm, scoop it into bowls and serve immediately.

Baked Pears with Cinnamon and Walnuts

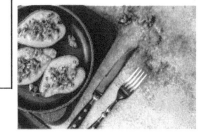

Prepping Time: 10 minutes
Cooking Time: 30 minutes
Portion Size: 4 servings

Nutritional Data: 120 calories
Protein: 1g | Fat: 4g
Carbohydrates: 21g | Fiber: 4g
Sugar: 15g | Sodium: 2 mg

Ingredients:
4 ripe pears, halved and cored
1/4 cup walnuts, chopped
2 tablespoons maple syrup or honey
1 teaspoon ground cinnamon
1/4 teaspoon ground nutmeg
1/2 teaspoon vanilla extract
Optional: Greek yogurt or whipped coconut cream for serving

Directions:
Preheat the oven to 375°F (190°C).
Place the pear halves in a baking dish, cut side up.
In a small bowl, mix the chopped walnuts, maple syrup (or honey), ground cinnamon, ground nutmeg, and vanilla extract.
Spoon the walnut mixture into the center of each pear half.
Bake in the preheated oven for 25-30 minutes, or until the pears are tender.
Serve warm, optionally topped with a dollop of Greek yogurt or whipped coconut cream.

No-Bake Peanut Butter Bars

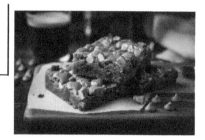

Prepping Time: 15 minutes
Cooking Time: 0 minutes
Portion Size: 12 bars

Nutritional Data: 230 calories
Protein: 6g | Fat: 16g
Carbohydrates: 18g | Fiber: 3g
Sugar: 8g | Sodium: 60 mg

Ingredients:
1 cup natural peanut butter
1/4 cup coconut oil, melted
1/4 cup maple syrup or honey
1 teaspoon vanilla extract
2 cups rolled oats
1/2 cup dark chocolate chips
1/4 cup chopped peanuts (optional)

Directions:
Line an 8x8 inch baking pan with parchment paper.
In a medium bowl, mix the peanut butter, melted coconut oil, maple syrup (or honey), and vanilla extract until smooth.
Add the rolled oats and stir until well combined. Press the mixture evenly into the prepared baking pan.
Melt the dark chocolate chips in a microwave-safe bowl or double boiler.
Spread the melted chocolate evenly over the peanut butter oat mixture. Sprinkle with chopped peanuts, if using.
Refrigerate for at least 2 hours, or until firm.
Once set, cut into 12 bars. Store in the refrigerator.

Mango and Coconut Ice Cream

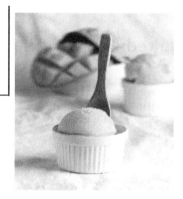

Prepping Time: 10 minutes
Cooking Time: 0 minutes
Portion Size: 4 servings

Nutritional Data: 210 calories
Protein: 2g | Fat: 12g
Carbohydrates: 27g | Fiber: 2g
Sugar: 23g | Sodium: 20 mg

Ingredients:
2 ripe mangoes, peeled and diced
1 can (14 oz) full-fat coconut milk
1/4 cup maple syrup or honey
1 teaspoon vanilla extract
Pinch of salt

Directions:
In a blender, combine the diced mangoes, coconut milk, maple syrup (or honey), vanilla extract, and a pinch of salt.
Blend until the mixture is smooth and creamy.
Pour the mixture into an ice cream maker and churn according to the manufacturer's instructions.
Transfer the churned ice cream into a lidded container and freeze for at least 4 hours, or until firm.
Scoop and serve. Enjoy your refreshing mango and coconut ice cream!

Chocolate Avocado Truffles

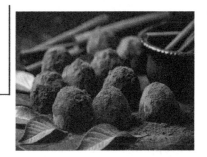

Prepping Time: 20 minutes
Cooking Time: 0 minutes
Portion Size: 12 truffles

Nutritional Data: 80 calories
Protein: 1g | Fat: 5g
Carbohydrates: 10g | Fiber: 3g
Sugar: 5g | Sodium: 10 mg

Ingredients:
1 large ripe avocado
1 cup dark chocolate chips (70% cocoa or higher)
1/4 cup unsweetened cocoa powder (for coating)
1/4 teaspoon vanilla extract
1 pinch sea salt
Optional: 1-2 tablespoons maple syrup or honey (for additional sweetness)

Directions:
Cut the avocado in half, remove the pit, and scoop out the flesh into a bowl. Mash the avocado until smooth and creamy.
Melt the dark chocolate chips in a double boiler or in the microwave in 30-second increments, stirring in between until completely melted.
Add the melted chocolate to the mashed avocado along with vanilla extract and a pinch of sea salt. If using, add maple syrup or honey for additional sweetness.
Mix until the ingredients are well combined and smooth.
Place the mixture in the refrigerator for about 30 minutes to firm up.
Once the mixture is firm, use a spoon to scoop out small portions and roll them into balls with your hands.
Roll each truffle in the unsweetened cocoa powder until evenly coated.
Store the truffles in the refrigerator until ready to serve.

Maple and Pecan Granola Bars

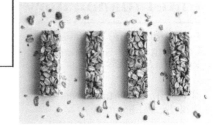

Prepping Time: 15 minutes
Cooking Time: 30 minutes
Portion Size: 12 bars

Nutritional Data: 220 calories
Protein: 4g | Fat: 12g
Carbohydrates: 24g | Fiber: 3g
Sugar: 10g | Sodium: 50 mg

Ingredients:

2 cups rolled oats
1 cup pecans, roughly chopped
1/2 cup almond butter
1/2 cup pure maple syrup
1/4 cup coconut oil
1/4 cup dried cranberries
1/4 cup unsweetened shredded coconut
1 teaspoon vanilla extract
1/2 teaspoon ground cinnamon
1/4 teaspoon sea salt

Directions:
Preheat the oven to 350°F (175°C). Line an 8x8-inch baking pan with parchment paper.
In a large mixing bowl, combine the rolled oats, chopped pecans, dried cranberries, shredded coconut, ground cinnamon, and sea salt. In a small saucepan over low heat, combine the almond butter, maple syrup, and coconut oil. Stir until the mixture is smooth and well combined. Remove from heat and stir in the vanilla extract. Pour the wet mixture over the dry ingredients and stir until everything is evenly coated. Transfer the mixture to the prepared baking pan and press it firmly into an even layer.
Bake in the preheated oven for 25-30 minutes, or until the edges are golden brown.
Allow the granola bars to cool completely in the pan before cutting them into bars.
Store in an airtight container at room temperature or in the refrigerator for up to one week.

BEVERAGES AND SMOOTHIES

Green Detox Smoothie with Spinach and Apple

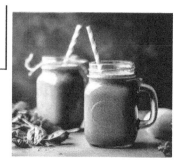

Prepping Time: 10 minutes
Cooking Time: 0 minutes
Portion Size: 2 servings

Nutritional Data: 110 calories
Protein: 2g | Fat: 2g
Carbohydrates: 25g | Fiber: 6g
Sugar: 13g | Sodium: 40 mg

Ingredients:
2 cups fresh spinach leaves
1 green apple, cored and chopped
1 banana
1/2 cucumber, peeled and chopped
1/2 lemon, juiced
1 tablespoon chia seeds
1 cup unsweetened almond milk (or any preferred plant-based milk)
1/2 cup water
Ice cubes (optional)

Directions:
In a blender, combine the spinach leaves, chopped green apple, banana, chopped cucumber, lemon juice, and chia seeds.
Add the almond milk and water.
Blend until smooth and creamy. Add ice cubes if a colder smoothie is desired.
Pour the smoothie into two glasses and serve immediately. Enjoy your nutritious Green Detox Smoothie!

Anti-Inflammatory Turmeric Golden Milk

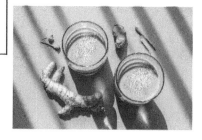

Prepping Time: 5 minutes
Cooking Time: 5 minutes
Portion Size: 2 servings

Nutritional Data: 70 calories
Protein: 1g | Fat: 2.5g
Carbohydrates: 11g | Fiber: 1g
Sugar: 7g | Sodium: 90 mg

Ingredients:

2 cups unsweetened almond milk (or any preferred plant-based milk)
1 teaspoon ground turmeric
1/2 teaspoon ground cinnamon
1/4 teaspoon ground ginger
1 tablespoon maple syrup or honey (optional)
1/4 teaspoon black pepper
1/2 teaspoon vanilla extract
Pinch of ground cloves (optional)

Directions:
In a small saucepan, combine the almond milk, ground turmeric, ground cinnamon, ground ginger, black pepper, and ground cloves (if using).
Heat the mixture over medium heat, stirring frequently to prevent burning.
Once the milk is hot but not boiling, remove it from the heat and stir in the maple syrup (or honey) and vanilla extract.
Pour the golden milk into two mugs and serve immediately. Enjoy your soothing Anti-Inflammatory Turmeric Golden Milk!

Berry Antioxidant Smoothie with Chia Seeds

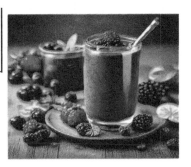

Prepping Time: 5 minutes
Cooking Time: 0 minutes
Portion Size: 2 servings

Nutritional Data: 150 calories
Protein: 3g | Fat: 3g
Carbohydrates: 31g | Fiber: 7g
Sugar: 15g | Sodium: 50 mg

Ingredients:
1 cup frozen mixed berries (blueberries, strawberries, raspberries)
1 banana
1 cup unsweetened almond milk (or any preferred plant-based milk)
1 tablespoon chia seeds
1 tablespoon honey or maple syrup (optional)
1/2 cup spinach (optional)
1/2 cup Greek yogurt (optional for extra creaminess)

Directions:
In a blender, combine the frozen mixed berries, banana, almond milk, chia seeds, and honey or maple syrup (if using).
Add spinach and Greek yogurt for additional nutrients and creaminess if desired.
Blend until smooth and creamy.
Pour the smoothie into two glasses and serve immediately. Enjoy your refreshing and nutritious Berry Antioxidant Smoothie with Chia Seeds!

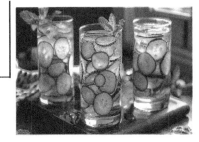

Cucumber and Mint Detox Water

Prepping Time: 10 minutes
Cooking Time: 0 minutes
Portion Size: 4 servings

Nutritional Data: 5 calories
Protein: 0g | Fat: 0g
Carbohydrates: 1g | Fiber: 0g
Sugar: 0g | Sodium: 5 mg

Ingredients:

1 cucumber, thinly sliced
10 fresh mint leaves
1 lemon, thinly sliced (optional)
8 cups water
Ice cubes (optional)

Directions:
In a large pitcher, combine cucumber slices, mint leaves, and lemon slices (if using).
Add water to the pitcher and stir gently.
Refrigerate for at least 1 hour to allow flavors to infuse.
Serve cold, adding ice cubes if desired.

Almond Butter and Banana Protein Smoothie

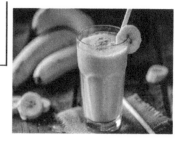

Prepping Time: 5 minutes
Cooking Time: 0 minutes
Portion Size: 2 servings

Nutritional Data: 300 calories
Protein: 15g | Fat: 12g
Carbohydrates: 35g | Fiber: 7g
Sugar: 14g | Sodium: 180 mg

Ingredients:

2 ripe bananas
2 tablespoons almond butter
1 cup almond milk (or any plant-based milk)
1 scoop vanilla protein powder
1 teaspoon chia seeds
1/2 teaspoon cinnamon (optional)
Ice cubes (optional)

Directions:
In a blender, combine bananas, almond butter, almond milk, protein powder, chia seeds, and cinnamon (if using).
Blend until smooth and creamy.
Add ice cubes if desired, and blend again until the ice is crushed and the smoothie is thick.
Pour into glasses and serve immediately.

Tropical Mango and Coconut Smoothie

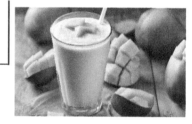

Prepping Time: 5 minutes
Cooking Time: 0 minutes
Portion Size: 2 servings

Nutritional Data: 200 calories
Protein: 2g | Fat: 8g
Carbohydrates: 32g | Fiber: 4g
Sugar: 24g | Sodium: 30 mg

Ingredients:

1 cup fresh or frozen mango chunks
1/2 cup coconut milk
1/2 cup coconut water
1 banana
1 tablespoon chia seeds (optional)
Ice cubes (optional)
Fresh mango slices for garnish (optional)

Directions:
In a blender, combine mango chunks, coconut milk, coconut water, banana, and chia seeds if using.
Blend until smooth and creamy.
Add ice cubes if desired and blend again until smooth.
Pour into glasses.
Garnish with fresh mango slices if using.
Serve immediately and enjoy!

Lavender and Lemon Infused Water

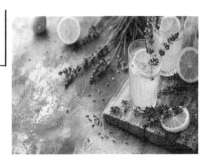

Prepping Time: 5 minutes
Cooking Time: 0 minutes
Portion Size: 4 servings

Nutritional Data: 5 calories
Protein: 0g | Fat: 0g
Carbohydrates: 1g | Fiber: 0g
Sugar: 0g | Sodium: 0 mg

Ingredients:

1 lemon, thinly sliced
1 tablespoon dried culinary lavender
4 cups water
Ice cubes (optional)
Fresh lavender sprigs for garnish (optional)

Directions:
In a large pitcher, combine lemon slices and dried lavender.
Pour water over the lemon and lavender mixture.
Stir well and let it sit in the refrigerator for at least 2 hours to infuse.
Add ice cubes if desired before serving.
Garnish with fresh lavender sprigs if using.
Serve chilled and enjoy your refreshing lavender and lemon infused water.

Avocado and Kale Power Smoothie

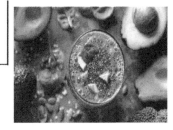

Prepping Time: 10 minutes
Cooking Time: 0 minutes
Portion Size: 2 servings

Nutritional Data: 250 calories
Protein: 3g | Fat: 18g
Carbohydrates: 22g | Fiber: 8g
Sugar: 10g | Sodium: 105 mg

Ingredients:

1 ripe avocado, peeled and pitted
1 cup kale leaves, stems removed
1 banana
1 cup unsweetened almond milk
1 tablespoon chia seeds
1 tablespoon honey (optional)
1/2 cup ice cubes (optional)

Directions:
In a blender, combine avocado, kale, banana, almond milk, chia seeds, and honey (if using).
Blend until smooth and creamy.
Add ice cubes if desired and blend again until smooth.
Pour into glasses and serve immediately.

Lemon and Ginger Immunity Boost Drink

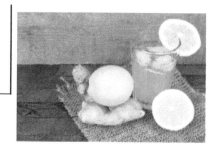

Prepping Time: 5 minutes
Cooking Time: 5 minutes
Portion Size: 2 servings

Nutritional Data: 20 calories
Protein: 0g | Fat: 0g
Carbohydrates: 5g | Fiber: 1g
Sugar: 4g | Sodium: 2 mg

Ingredients:

2 cups water
1 lemon, juiced
1-inch piece of fresh ginger, peeled and sliced
1 tablespoon honey (optional)
1/2 teaspoon turmeric (optional)

Directions:
In a small saucepan, bring the water to a boil.
Add the sliced ginger to the boiling water and reduce the heat. Let it simmer for 5 minutes.
Remove the saucepan from heat and let it cool slightly.
Stir in the lemon juice and honey (if using). Add turmeric for extra anti-inflammatory benefits, if desired.
Strain the drink into a glass and serve warm.

Watermelon and Basil Cooler

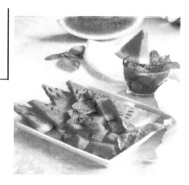

Prepping Time: 10 minutes
Cooking Time: 0 minutes
Portion Size: 4 servings

Nutritional Data: 50 calories
Protein: 1g | Fat: 0g
Carbohydrates: 12g | Fiber: 1g
Sugar: 10g | Sodium: 2 mg

Ingredients:

4 cups watermelon, cubed and deseeded
1/4 cup fresh basil leaves
Juice of 1 lime
1 tablespoon honey (optional)
Ice cubes

Directions:
In a blender, combine the watermelon cubes, basil leaves, lime juice, and honey (if using).
Blend until smooth.
Pour the mixture through a fine mesh strainer into a pitcher to remove the pulp.
Serve the cooler over ice cubes in glasses and enjoy immediately.

Spirulina and Pineapple Superfood Smoothie

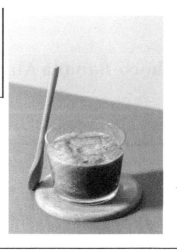

Prepping Time: 5 minutes
Cooking Time: 0 minutes
Portion Size: 2 servings

Nutritional Data: 180 calories
Protein: 3g | Fat: 2g
Carbohydrates: 40g | Fiber: 7g
Sugar: 18g | Sodium: 75 mg

Ingredients:

1 cup fresh pineapple chunks
1 banana
1 cup spinach leaves
1 teaspoon spirulina powder
1 tablespoon chia seeds
1 cup coconut water
1/2 cup ice cubes

Directions:
In a blender, combine the pineapple chunks, banana, spinach leaves, spirulina powder, chia seeds, coconut water, and ice cubes.
Blend until smooth and creamy.
Pour the smoothie into glasses and serve immediately.

Carrot and Orange Refreshing Juice

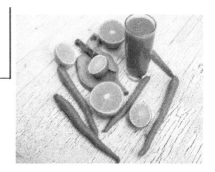

Prepping Time: 10 minutes
Cooking Time: 0 minutes
Portion Size: 2 servings

Nutritional Data: 110 calories
Protein: 2g | Fat: 0.5g
Carbohydrates: 26g | Fiber: 6g
Sugar: 18g | Sodium: 40 mg

Ingredients:

4 large carrots, peeled and chopped
2 large oranges, peeled and segmented
1 tablespoon fresh lemon juice
1 teaspoon fresh ginger, grated
1 cup cold water
Ice cubes (optional)

Directions:
In a blender, combine the chopped carrots, orange segments, fresh lemon juice, grated ginger, and cold water.
Blend until smooth.
Strain the juice through a fine-mesh sieve or cheesecloth to remove the pulp, if desired.
Pour the juice into glasses over ice cubes, if using.
Serve immediately and enjoy the refreshing drink.

Choco-Banana Almond Smoothie

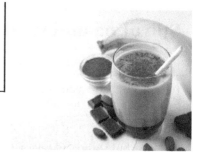

Prepping Time: 5 minutes
Cooking Time: 0 minutes
Portion Size: 2 servings

Nutritional Data: 250 calories
Protein: 6g | Fat: 11g
Carbohydrates: 35g | Fiber: 8g
Sugar: 15g | Sodium: 150 mg

Ingredients:

2 ripe bananas
2 tablespoons almond butter
1 tablespoon unsweetened cocoa powder
1 cup unsweetened almond milk
1 tablespoon chia seeds
1 teaspoon vanilla extract
Ice cubes (optional)

Directions:
In a blender, combine the ripe bananas, almond butter, unsweetened cocoa powder, unsweetened almond milk, chia seeds, and vanilla extract.
Blend until smooth and creamy.
Add ice cubes if you prefer a colder, thicker smoothie.
Pour into glasses and serve immediately.

Apple Cider Vinegar Detox Drink

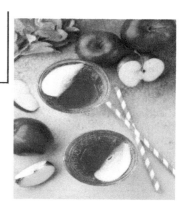

Prepping Time: 5 minutes
Cooking Time: 0 minutes
Portion Size: 1 serving

Nutritional Data: 25 calories
Protein: 0g | Fat: 0g
Carbohydrates: 6g | Fiber: 0.5g
Sugar: 5g | Sodium: 5 mg

Ingredients:

1 cup water (warm or cold)
1 tablespoon apple cider vinegar
1 tablespoon lemon juice
1/2 teaspoon ground cinnamon
1 tablespoon honey (optional)
1/2 teaspoon grated ginger (optional)

Directions:
In a glass, combine the water, apple cider vinegar, lemon juice, and ground cinnamon.
Stir well until the ingredients are fully mixed.
Add honey and grated ginger if desired, and stir until dissolved.
Drink immediately for best results.

Blueberry and Oat Breakfast Smoothie

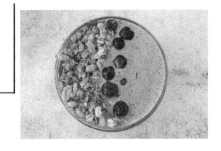

Prepping Time: 5 minutes
Cooking Time: 0 minutes
Portion Size: 2 servings

Nutritional Data: 230 calories
Protein: 5g | Fat: 4g
Carbohydrates: 45g | Fiber: 7g
Sugar: 15g | Sodium: 80 mg

Ingredients:

1 cup fresh or frozen blueberries
1 banana
1/2 cup rolled oats
1 cup almond milk (or any plant-based milk)
1 tablespoon chia seeds
1 tablespoon honey or maple syrup (optional)
1/2 teaspoon vanilla extract

Directions:
In a blender, combine the blueberries, banana, rolled oats, almond milk, chia seeds, honey or maple syrup (if using), and vanilla extract.
Blend until smooth and creamy.
Pour into glasses and serve immediately. Enjoy your nutritious Blueberry and Oat Breakfast Smoothie!

Papaya and Lime Digestive Aid Smoothie

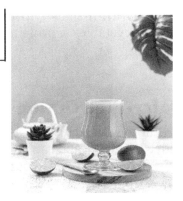

Prepping Time: 10 minutes
Cooking Time: 0 minutes
Portion Size: 2 servings

Nutritional Data: 180 calories
Protein: 4g | Fat: 2g
Carbohydrates: 38g | Fiber: 4g
Sugar: 26g | Sodium: 50 mg

Ingredients:

1 ripe papaya, peeled, seeded, and chopped
Juice of 1 lime
1 cup coconut water
1/2 cup Greek yogurt (optional for added creaminess)
1 tablespoon honey or maple syrup (optional)
1/2 teaspoon grated fresh ginger

Directions:
In a blender, combine the chopped papaya, lime juice, coconut water, Greek yogurt (if using), honey or maple syrup (if using), and grated fresh ginger.
Blend until smooth and creamy.
Pour into glasses and serve immediately. Enjoy your refreshing and digestive-aiding Papaya and Lime Smoothie!

SPECIAL DIETS AND CONSIDERATIONS

In today's diverse culinary landscape, adapting recipes to meet various dietary needs is essential. Whether due to allergies, intolerances, or personal preferences, having flexible recipes that can be easily modified ensures that everyone can enjoy healthy, delicious meals. The importance of whole, natural foods, making it straightforward to adapt recipes to be gluten-free, dairy-free, vegetarian, and more. This chapter provides guidelines and tips for adjusting recipes to accommodate different dietary requirements.

Gluten-Free Options

Gluten intolerance and celiac disease require strict adherence to a gluten-free diet. Fortunately, many whole foods and natural ingredients are naturally gluten-free, making adaptation easier.

Key Substitutes:
- Flours: Replace wheat flour with almond flour, coconut flour, rice flour, or gluten-free oat flour.
- Grains: Use quinoa, rice, millet, and buckwheat instead of wheat, barley, or rye.
- Pasta: Opt for pasta made from rice, corn, quinoa, or lentils.

→ **Recipe Adaptation Example**:
- *Gluten-Free Quinoa Salad*: Replace couscous or bulgur with cooked quinoa. Add your favorite vegetables, a protein source like chickpeas, and dress with olive oil and lemon juice.

Dairy-Free Options

For those with lactose intolerance or a dairy allergy, or who prefer a vegan diet, dairy-free alternatives are widely available and can be incorporated into most recipes.

Key Substitutes:
- Milk: Use almond milk, soy milk, coconut milk, or oat milk.
- Cheese: Substitute dairy cheese with cashew cheese, almond cheese, or nutritional yeast for a cheesy flavor.
- Butter: Replace butter with coconut oil, olive oil, or vegan butter.

→ **Recipe Adaptation Example**:
- *Dairy-Free Smoothie*: Blend your favorite fruits with almond milk or coconut milk, adding a tablespoon of chia seeds for extra nutrition.

Vegetarian Options

Vegetarian diets exclude meat but can include a variety of other nutrient-rich foods. Adapting recipes to be vegetarian involves replacing meat with plant-based proteins.

Key Substitutes:
- Meat: Use tofu, tempeh, seitan, lentils, beans, or chickpeas.
- Broth: Replace chicken or beef broth with vegetable broth.

→ Recipe Adaptation Example:
- *Vegetarian Lentil Soup*: Substitute ground beef with lentils and use vegetable broth instead of chicken broth. Add plenty of vegetables and spices for a hearty, nutritious soup.

Adjusting Recipes for Allergies and Intolerances

When adjusting recipes for allergies and intolerances, it's essential to identify safe substitutes that maintain the dish's flavor and texture. Below are strategies for common allergens.

Nut Allergies:
- Substitute Nuts: Use seeds such as sunflower seeds or pumpkin seeds in place of nuts in recipes.
- Nut Butters: Replace almond or peanut butter with sunflower seed butter or tahini.

Soy Allergies:
- Substitute Soy Sauce: Use coconut aminos or tamari (gluten-free soy sauce) if not avoiding gluten.
- Replace Tofu/Tempeh: Use chickpeas, lentils, or other legumes as a protein source.

Egg Allergies:
- Egg Substitutes: Use flaxseed meal or chia seeds mixed with water (1 tablespoon seeds + 3 tablespoons water) to replace eggs in baking. Applesauce or mashed bananas can also work in some recipes.

→ Recipe Adaptation Example:

- ***Nut-Free Energy Balls***: Replace nuts with sunflower seeds and use sunflower seed butter instead of almond butter. Combine with dates, oats, and cocoa powder for a delicious snack.

Adapting recipes to meet various dietary needs ensures inclusivity and health for everyone. By understanding and implementing key substitutions, you can modify any recipe to be gluten-free, dairy-free, vegetarian, or free of other allergens. Focusing on whole, natural foods makes it easier to create flexible, nutritious, and delicious meals suitable for all dietary requirements.

4 WEEK MEAL PLAN

Below is a 4-week meal plan based on the recipes provided above, ensuring a variety of nutrient-dense, and balanced meals. Each week includes breakfast, lunch, dinner, and snack options.

WEEK 1

DAY	MONDAY	TUESDAY	WEDNESDAY	THURSDAY	FRIDAY	SATURDAY	SUNDAY
Breakfast	Green Goddess Smoothie Bowl (p.16)	Quinoa and Berry Breakfast Parfait (p.17)	Apple Cinnamon Quinoa Breakfast Bake (p.21)	Coconut and Mango Chia Seed Pudding (p.20)	Protein-Packed Overnight Chia Pudding (p.16)	Veggie-Loaded Chickpea Breakfast Wrap (p.18)	Hearty Buckwheat Porridge with Nuts and Seeds (p.18)
Lunch	Quinoa and Kale Salad with Lemon-Tahini Dressing (p.26)	Chickpea and Avocado Stuffed Bell Peppers (p.26)	Grilled Vegetable and Hummus Wrap (p.27)	Lentil and Spinach Soup with Turmeric (p.27)	Turmeric-Spiced Lentil and Rice Pilaf (p.35)	Spaghetti Squash with Pesto and Cherry Tomatoes (p.30)	Rainbow Veggie Buddha Bowl (p.29)
Dinner	Roasted Vegetable and Quinoa Stuffed Peppers (p.37)	Lentil and Sweet Potato Shepherd's Pie (p.37)	Cauliflower Steak with Chimichurri Sauce (p.38)	Spicy Chickpea and Spinach Curry (p.38)	Baked Salmon with Lemon-Dill Quinoa (p.39)	Zucchini Lasagna with Cashew Ricotta (p.39)	Eggplant and Mushroom Stir-Fry with Brown Rice (p.40)
Snack options	Spicy Roasted Chickpeas (p.45)	Raw Energy Balls with Dates and Nuts (p.48)	Fresh Veggie Spring Rolls with Almond Sauce (p.45)	Quinoa and Black Bean Salad (p.46)	Edamame with Sea Salt and Lemon (p.51)	Cabbage and Carrot Sauerkraut (p.50)	Turmeric-Spiced Roasted Cauliflower (p.46)

Feel free to adjust the meal plan to fit your preferences and dietary needs. Enjoy your meals!

WEEK 2

DAY	MONDAY	TUESDAY	WEDNESDAY	THURSDAY	FRIDAY	SATURDAY	SUNDAY
Breakfast	Tropical Green Smoothie with Spirulina (p.21)	Almond Butter and Banana Breakfast Bowl (p.25)	Blueberry Almond Overnight Oats (p.19)	Spinach and Avocado Power Smoothie (p.17)	Berry and Blast Smoothie with Chia Seeds (p.23)	Savory Quinoa and Veggie Breakfast Boal (p.19)	Zucchini and Carrot Breakfast Muffins (p.22)
Lunch	Sweet Potato and Black Bean Burrito Bowl (p.31)	Zucchini Noodles with Avocado Basil Pesto (p.31)	Broccoli and Almond Stir-Fry with Brown Rice (p.36)	Hearty Minestrone Soup with Quinoa (p.32)	Greek Salad with Quinoa and Chickpeas (p.33)	Butternut Squash and Lentil Stew (p.34)	Fresh Spring Rolls with Peanut Dipping Sauce (p.34)
Dinner	Butternut Squash and Black Bean Enchiladas (p.40)	Herb-Crusted Tofu with Roasted Brussels Sprouts (p.41)	Eggplant and Mushroom Stir-Fry with Brown Rice (p. 40)	Spinach and Mushroom Stuffed Portobello Mushrooms (p.44)	Spaghetti with Zucchini Noodles and Pesto (p.42)	Mediterranean Chickpea and Spinach Sauté (p.41)	Quinoa and Vegetable Stuffed Cabbage Rolls (p.42)
Snack options	Garlic and Herb Hummus with Carrot Sticks (p.47)	Cabbage and Carrot Sauerkraut (p.50)	Zucchini Fritters with Yogurt Dip (p.47)	Crispy Baked Tofu Bites (p.48)	Raw Energy Balls with Dates and Nuts (p.48)	Broccoli and Walnut Salad (p.49)	Tomato and Basil Bruschetta on Whole Grain Bread (p.49)

WEEK 3

DAY	MONDAY	TUESDAY	WEDNESDAY	THURSDAY	FRIDAY	SATURDAY	SUNDAY
Breakfast	Smashed Chickpea and Avocado (p.24)	Blueberry Almond Overnight Oats (p.19)	Coconut and Mango Chia Seed Pudding (p.20)	Banana Walnut Overnight Oats (p.22)	Kale and Sweet Potato Breakfast Hash (p.20)	Herbed Avocado and Tomato Breakfast Toast (p.23)	Protein-Packed Overnight Chia Pudding (p.16)
Lunch	Spaghetti Squash with Pesto and Cherry Tomatoes (p.30)	Veggie-Pached Quinoa Patties with Avocad Sauce (p.35)	Turmeric-Spiced Lentil and Rice Pilaf (p.35)	Roasted Beet and Arugula Salad with Walnuts (p.36)	Broccoli and Almond Stir-Fry with Brown Rice (p.36)	Mixed Bean Salad with Fresh Herbs (p.30)	Greek Salad with Quinoa and Chickpeas (p.33)
Dinner	Turmeric and Ginger Lentil Soup (p.43)	Zucchini Lasagna with Cashew Ricotta (p.39)	Moroccan-Spiced Vegetable Tagine (p.43)	Spicy Chickpea and Spinach Curry (p.38)	Spinach and Mushroom Stuffed Portobello Mushrooms (p.44)	Baked Salmon with Lemon-Dill Quinoa (p.39)	Quinoa and Vegetable Stuffed Cabbage Rolls (p.42)
Snack options	Garlic and Herb Hummus with Carrot Sticks (p.47)	Avocado and Lime Guacamole with Veggie Chips (p.50)	Cabbage and Carrot Sauerkraut (p.50)	Broccoli and Walnut Salad (p.49)	Marinated Olives with Lemon and Thyme (p.51)	Edamame with Sea Salt and Lemon (p.51)	Raw Energy Balls with Dates and Nuts (p.48)

WEEK 4

DAY	MONDAY	TUESDAY	WEDNESDAY	THURSDAY	FRIDAY	SATURDAY	SUNDAY
Breakfast	Green Goddes Smoothie Bowl (p.16)	Pumpkin Spice Chia Pudding (p.24)	Superfood Acai Bowl with Fresh Berries (p.25)	Berry Blast Smoothie with Chia Seeds (p.23)	Almond Butter and Banana Breakfast Bowl (p.25)	Protein-Pached Overnight Chia Pudding (p.16)	Tropical Green Smoothie with Spirulina (p.21)
Lunch	Stuffed Portobello Mushrooms with Spinach and Feta (p.33)	Rainbow Veggie Buddha Bowl (p.29)	Chickpea and Avocado Stuffed Bell Peppers (p.26)	Grilled Vegetable and Hummus Wrap (p.27)	Lentil and Spinach Soup with Turmeric (p.27)	Cauliflower Rice Stir-Fry with Tofu (p.32)	Zucchini Noodles with Avocado Basil Pesto (p.31)
Dinner	Herb-Crusted Tofu with Roasted Brussels Sprouts (p.41)	Mixed Bean Salad with Fresh Herbs (p.44)	Cauliflower Rice Stir-Fry with Tofu (p.45)	Cauliflower Steak with Chimichurri Sauce (p.38)	Lentil and Sweet Potato Shepherd's Pie (p.37)	Baked Salmon with Lemon-Dill Quinoa (p.39)	Spicy Chickpea and Spinach Curry (p.38)
Snack options	Avocaado and Lime Guacamole with Veggie Chips (p.50)	Fresh Veggie Spring Rolls with Almond Sauce (p.45)	Zucchini Fritters with Yogurt Dip (p.47)	Spicy Roasted Chickpeas (p.45)	Crispy Baked Tofu Bites (p.48)	Tomato and Basil Bruschetta on Whole Grain Bread (p.49)	Marinated Olives with Lemon and Thyme (p.51)

CONCLUSIONS

Thank you for joining me on this journey towards optimal health with this cookbook." Through Anti-Inflammatory Diet principles, I have explored the transformative power of a balanced, nutrient-rich diet composed of whole, natural foods.

This book is designed to provide you with practical, delicious, and adaptable recipes that support your health goals. By focusing on whole foods and natural ingredients, you are giving your body the best possible foundation for health and well-being. The variety of recipes ensures you get a balance of essential nutrients, while also catering to different dietary needs with gluten-free, dairy-free, and vegetarian options.

My goal has been to make healthy eating accessible and enjoyable, encouraging you to embrace a lifestyle that supports your body's natural healing processes.

Your commitment to nourishing your body with wholesome foods is a powerful step towards lasting health.

Thank you for reading and allowing me to be part of your journey.

If you found this book helpful, please leave an honest review on Amazon. Your feedback is invaluable to me and will help others on their wellness journey.

Thank you, and here's to your health and happiness!

SCAN HERE TO PRINT

THE QUICK REFERENCE GUIDES:

OR COPY AND PASTE THE URL:

https://drive.google.com/file/d/1A7ICDeRgWidHZfxlAGhcq_
W9Oql1wR9G/view?usp=drive_link

THE GROCERY LIST:

OR COPY AND PASTE THE URL:

https://drive.google.com/file/d/1qnG1Mvt4V9NcPGtAJ_6wY8
54zR19Kwny/view?usp=drive_link

Made in the USA
Las Vegas, NV
24 October 2024

10428576R00044